The World Anti-Doping

Following the recent doping scandals that have brought the highest echelons of international sport into disrepute, this book examines the elitism at the core of the World Anti-Doping Agency and considers how the current World Anti-Doping Code might be restructured.

Analyzing the correlation between the commodification of sports and doping, and the role WADA plays in this context, it takes into consideration the perspectives of non-elite athletes as well as athletes from developing countries which have previously been excluded from the anti-doping discourse. It offers recommendations for improving the coordination and implementation of the World Anti-Doping Code and argues for the creation of a more inclusive anti-doping regime.

This is an important resource for students of sports law, sports management and sports ethics, as well as vital reading for sports administrators, sports sociologists, sports policy makers, sports lawyers and arbitrators, as well as athletes themselves.

Lovely Dasgupta is Assistant Professor of Law at the West Bengal National University of Juridical Sciences, India, with particular interests in Sports Law, Competition Law and Contract Law. She became one of the pioneers in the field of studying and researching on Sports Law from an Indian perspective and was one of the first from the Indian legal fraternity to develop and teach the subject called Sports Law. She has appeared in interviews aired on the BBC about the doping scenario in India and Women's Cricket in India.

Routledge Research in Sport, Culture and Society

For more information about this series, please visit: www.routledge.com/sport/series/RRSCS

The World Anti-Doping Code

Fit for Purpose?

Lovely Dasgupta

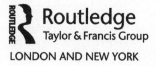

Routledge
Taylor & Francis Group

LONDON AND NEW YORK

First published 2019 by Routledge

2 Park Square, Milton Park, Abingdon, Oxon, OX14 4RN
605 Third Avenue, New York, NY 10017

Routledge is an imprint of the Taylor & Francis Group, an informa business

First issued in paperback 2020

British Library Cataloguing-in-Publication Data
A catalogue record for this book is available from the British Library

Library of Congress Cataloging-in-Publication Data
A catalog record for this book has been requested

ISBN: 978-1-138-49747-4 (hbk)
ISBN: 978-0-367-72956-1 (pbk)

Typeset in Goudy
by Apex CoVantage, LLC

Contents

Preface

Pierre de Coubertin can be regarded as the inspiration behind the current anti-doping regime, and that is where the entire pretense of the system lies. It is essentially a false start and a flawed foundation on which World Anti-Doping Agency (WADA) is made to stand. WADA, however, is not in isolation, because it mirrors the duplicity of all the International Federations as well as the International Olympic Committee. All these organizations propagate a philosophy rooted in the so-called purity of sport. This ignores the reality of professionals having overtaken amateurs in all sports. This also ignores the fact that, like all professionals, athletes seek the highest level of incentives through winning performances. Hence it ignores that, like all true professionals, athletes seek glory but with a curriculum vitae that mirrors their success. This double-faced approach of the sporting world is evident from the fact that despite innumerable scandals and allegations of ongoing, widespread doping, the Tour de France continues to be promoted as the ultimate test of human endurance against the challenges thrown by nature. This is a chimera created by sports administrators with the help of the media. It plays upon the idealism that sports are meant to be a test of pure human skill. The question that comes to mind at this juncture is, what is purity? Human skill needs enhancement through training and other assistance. If this is the case, then why create the myth of sport being something to be revered? The very fact that the International Olympic Committee contracts with host cities to protect its intellectual property undermines all talk about sport being free from commercial exploits. The zillion-dollar television contracts that the International Federations sign also shatter the myth of sport being about amateurs. This book intervenes by pointing out that, to date, WADA has operated through the process of mythification of sport. In my opinion, WADA is also in a state of denial and continues to ignore the history relating to performance-enhancing drugs in sport. This is problematic because the current anti-doping regime seeks to prescribe an anti-doping solution without undertaking a thorough and deep diagnosis of the reasons for doping.

The promotion of elitism in sports is the offshoot of commercialization and commodification of sports. It is also evident in the reality of professionalism in the field of sports. Historically, sports were played by professionals in a manner quite contrary to the idea of purity and amateurism. They were impacted by the political and cultural developments of their time, and amateurism was not an ideal to which everyone aspired. The point then is that acceptance of professionalism within sports or a professional sportsperson as a reality is not derogatory. This book argues for coming out of the Coubertin fixation and taking a more universal look towards the usage of drugs in sports. The recognition of sports as a source of livelihood ensures that we need, while formulating the rules and World Anti-Doping Code (the Code), to ensure the observance of basic rights. Over the years, WADA has furnished arguments in support of the Code and its revisions. The approach has been to divide the sporting world into two halves: one for doping and one against doping. This book intervenes by raising the question of why it has to be an either-or situation. If we acknowledge that sportspersons are professionals, then their usage of both performance-enhancing drugs and performance-enhancing technology ought to be treated in the same manner. This book questions the methodology adopted in the WADA Code, arguing that it inhibits rather than promotes professionalism in sport.

Another reason why WADA needs to re-orient itself stems from the findings of the two Independent Commission reports submitted by Richard Pound. Richard H. McLaren, O.C., appointed as the independent person to submit reports on doping in the Sochi Winter Olympics, also has highlighted issues pertaining to the existing anti-doping programme. Interestingly all the provisions within the WADA Code give an impression of a stringent anti-doping regime. However, violation of these provisions, with the collusion of sports officials, indicates not only a flawed implementation by WADA, but also the limitations of WADA as a dope regulator. This calls for WADA to take itself less seriously and to formulate out-of-the-box ideas to ensure better execution of its mandate. Importantly, WADA's autonomy needs to be re-visited, with perhaps better coordination with state actors. Furthermore, the current structure has not given up the philosophical ideology with which it started under the 2004 WADA Code. This is problematic in view of the doping scandals that have occurred since then. This book intervenes to argue that there needs to be a revision of the underlying philosophical positions taken with respect to anti-doping regulations. This re-examination has to be both in terms of strict liability as well as autonomy of the sports institutions. This book also brings forth the inherent conflict that is created when WADA insists on its autonomy on the one hand and yet propagates strict liability on the other. The danger is lack of accountability while upstaging of athletes' rights.

The objectives of this book are fivefold:

1   There is a divide between the elite versus the non-elite within the world of sports, and the current anti-doping regulations are geared towards protecting the interests of the elite.
2   The elite, in this book are the rich, famous and powerful sportspersons able to dictate the terms on which the rules will apply and the sanctions that will be imposed under the current anti-doping regime.

3   The concept of sports autonomy is detrimental to an equitable anti-doping regime because it does not permit accountability or deal with the concerns of access to justice.
4   The strict liability philosophy undermines all attempts at making sports institutions like WADA responsive to the demands of developing inclusive anti-doping regulations.
5   The private–public partnership in terms of coordination with state fact-finding agencies needs to be encouraged and institutionalized within a WADA-run anti-doping regime.

In the process, this book:

1   Brings forth the perspectives of non-elite athletes, overcoming the current predominance of an elite perspective of the WADA Code.
2   Re-defines the understanding of elitism in sport by widening the concept to include high-performing athletes from developing countries or poor backgrounds.
3   Underlines the need for an intergovernmental framework to coordinate with WADA for proper investigations and better implementation.
4   Advocates for the institutionalization of legal aid and technology transfer by WADA to less developed regions for better anti-doping education and access to justice.
5   Urges the adoption of a soft strict-liability approach, suited to the needs of the sporting world and enabling development of a nuanced anti-doping detection mechanism.

From the first to the fifth chapter, this book argues for WADA to be inclusive and to accommodate the perspectives of non-elite athletes from developing countries. Chapter 1 traces the historical roots and justification of the current anti-doping regime. Chapter 2 examines the Russian doping scandal, which has proven to be the biggest challenge for WADA to date. The chapter presents the progression of the scandal and the reaction of the sport authorities and governing bosses, identifying various instances of WADA's pro-elite approach. Against this background, Chapter 3 looks into various provisions of the WADA Code that promote a pro-elite approach. The problem is that satisfying the standards required in the provisions requires lots of money, and many non-elite athletes lack the means to defend their cases. Chapter 4 goes into detail about the current situation for non-elite athletes from developing countries. Most of these non-elite athletes are not conversant with the sophisticated doping practices that elite athletes use to con the system, and, as a result, non-elite athletes from developing countries are more likely to be caught. Further, their lack of resources affects their ability to negotiate the WADA system. Thus, they end up being the voiceless constituents of sports. Chapter 5 looks into the possible intervention that can result in a fairer system for all.

Chapter 1

The anti-doping narrative

A case of self-legitimization

Introduction

This chapter looks into the world of sport before the implementation of WADA as well as the scandals that ultimately led to WADA. The chapter will examine the deliberations that took place at the International Convention Against Doping in Sport that was organized by UNESCO. The document that resulted from this Convention will be analysed to highlight the interaction between governmental and non-governmental bodies on the issue of doping in sport. The Convention legitimized the argument of an existing consensus on adopting strict anti-doping measures, but it remains to be seen what the role of the state is in implementing and ensuring effective anti-doping measures. This leads to the inevitable question of the autonomy that WADA was proposed to be given as compared to the autonomy that WADA ought to have been given. The other issue is with respect to the role that sports governing bodies were ready to concede in favour of the state governments for the purpose of enforcing anti-doping measures. Most importantly, this chapter investigates the real intent for developing a consensus on adopting anti-doping regulations viz. to stop trafficking in drugs or to protect health or to prevent performance enhancement. If the real agenda was to prevent large-scale scams, then trafficking definitely is one of the concerns. However, the question that arises is whether the sports governing bodies are well enough equipped and have the necessary jurisdiction to prevent trafficking. If not, then the only other entity that can prevent trafficking is the state. If the state is to play a major role in stopping trafficking, then a global intergovernmental body is needed to enforce anti-doping measures. If the real agenda is to protect health through anti-doping measures, then the state appears to be the aptest entity to enforce such measures. After all, public health policies are to be framed by the state, and there is no argument that sportspersons have different health concerns than ordinary people. If performance enhancement is the sole goal of anti-doping measures, then questions are bound to arise in categorizing legitimate performance enhancement techniques vis-à-vis illegitimate performance enhancement techniques. Using the "spirit of sport" argument as justifying the current anti-doping regime is the other point that needs to be understood.

The spirit of sport argument invokes the ideals of amateurism and overlooks the reality of professionalism. Hence, the justification of the WADA Code is coming from within the system and in the absence of any external parameters. It is a case of self-legitimization. The extent of this process of self-affirmation without debating the issues of autonomy, the intent of anti-doping philosophy or the validity of the concept of spirit of sport are the topics of discussion in this chapter. The first chapter thus maps all the aspects of the debate to point out the nature of the existing anti-doping regime.

Late beginning! Flip-flop on psychotropic performance enhancers

In 1968 the International Olympic Committee (IOC) officially banned doping.[1] The International Association of Athletics Federation (IAAF)[2] was the first sports federation to ban performance-enhancing drugs in 1928.[3] Considering that the modern Olympics started in 1896,[4] this late vilification of performance-enhancing drugs (PEDs) appears to be an afterthought. Documented literature on the history of doping indicates that the use of PEDs in modern sports was an accepted fact.[5] One of the most celebrated examples of the use of PEDs in sports is that of American marathon runner Thomas J. Hicks.[6] In the official report of the 1904 Olympics, prepared by Charles Lucas, there is a detailed account of the Hicks case.[7] Charles Lucas, who was also one of the officials in charge of Hicks, reported that Hicks was administered small doses of sulphate of strychnine.[8] This dosage was given at intervals whenever Lucas and his colleagues felt that Hicks would collapse. Hicks was given one-sixtieth of a grain of sulphate of strychnine along with the white of one egg when he was seven miles away from the stadium.[9] Again, when Hicks had crossed twenty miles and was starting to look ashen, one-sixtieth grain of strychnine was administered to him along with two

1 Wayne Wilson and Edward Derse (ed.), *Doping in Elite Sport-the Politics of Drugs in the Olympic Movement* (Human Kinetics Publishers, 2001)
2 Formerly known as International Amateur Athletic Federation
3 Hand Book of the International Amateur Athletic Federation, 1927–28, Section 13 and Section 22 www.iaaf.org/news/news/a-piece-of-anti-doping-history-iaaf-handbook (accessed 1 February 2018)
4 Athens 1896 www.olympic.org/athens-1896 (accessed 1 February 2018)
5 Annette Greenhow, "Drug Use in Sport: What's Changed?" (2010), 16 (2) *The National Legal Eagle* http://epublications.bond.edu.au/cgi/viewcontent.cgi?article=1152&context=nle (accessed 1 February 2018)
6 Karen Abbott, "The 1904 Olympic Marathon May Have Been the Strangest Ever" (2012) Smithsonian.com www.smithsonianmag.com/history/the-1904-olympic-marathon-may-have-been-the-strangest-ever-14910747/ (accessed 1 February 2018)
7 Charles J. P. Lucas, *The Olympic Games-1904* (St. Louis, MO, Woodward & Tiernan Printing Co., 1905) http://library.la84.org/6oic/OfficialReports/1904/1904lucas.pdf (accessed 2 February 2018)
8 Ibid 50
9 Ibid 52

eggs and a sip of brandy.[10] This description, being part of the official record of the 1904 Olympics, clearly indicates the acceptability of the practice of using psychotropic performance enhancers/PEDs. This chemically aided win was not looked down upon or derided. On the contrary, it was celebrated as an honest win.[11] This incident within sports merely mirrors the then-prevailing societal attitude in the West towards psychotropic substance.[12] The representation of drug use in popular Western culture (e.g. songs of the 1930s) substantiate this condescending attitude.[13] A clear instance of this is the song "Wacky Dust" by Ella Fitzgerald, in which she exalts the use of cocaine.[14]

In sports like cycling, horse racing,[15] swimming, sprinting, long distance running etc., the use of PEDs was very common.[16] The use of these psychotropic performance enhancers was done openly and without secrecy.[17] Similarly, there have been instances of the use of PEDs in professional football.[18] For instance during the 1924–25 FA Cup, Arsenal players used stimulants in their match against West Ham United.[19] Hence, there appeared to be no inherent bias in the West against the use of psychotropic drugs in sports.[20] Further, the use of different PEDs in sports was also accelerated by the growth of sports science.[21] Sport performance provided an important field of study to understand human biology.[22] Thus, early attempts to establish anti-doping laws/regulations need to be rationalized on parameters other than moralistic aversion to the use of PEDs. Historical accounts of the origins of anti-doping regulations in sport are rooted in concerns with

10 Ibid 53
11 Ibid 60
12 Susan Boyd, "Pleasure and Pain-representations of Illegal Drug Consumption, Addiction and Trafficking in Music, Film and Video" in Suzanne Fraser and David Moore (eds.), *The Drug Effect: Health, Crime and Society* (Cambridge University Press, 2011)
13 Ibid. Some examples of such representation in the popular culture are Cab Calloway, "The Reefer Man (Original)" www.youtube.com/watch?v=svoSSdsNhtA; Weed Smoker's Dream, "Harlem Hamfats" www.youtube.com/watch?v=uyjW8FTGxbI; Ella Fitzgerald, "Wacky Dust" www.youtube.com/watch?v=RjRcKq38-IY (accessed 7 February 2018)
14 Ibid
15 Mark Johnson, *Spitting in the Soup-inside the Dirty Game of Doping in Sports* (VeloPress 2016)
16 Charles E. Yesalis and Michael S. Bahrke, "History of Doping in Sport" (2002) 24 (1) *International Sports Studies* http://library.la84.org/SportsLibrary/ISS/ISS2401/ISS2401e.pdf (accessed 8 February 2018)
17 Ibid 46
18 I Waddington, D Malcolm, M Roderick and R Naik, "Drug use in English Professional Football" (2005) 39 (18) *British Journal of Sports Medicine* www.bjsportmed.com/cgi/content/full/39/4/e18; doi: 10.1136/bjsm.2004.012468 (accessed 7 February 2018)
19 Bernard Joy, *Forward, Arsenal! The First Detailed History of Arsenal Football Club 1886–1953* (GCR Books, 2009)
20 Ian Ritchie, "Cops and Robbers? The Roots of Anti-Doping Policies in Olympic Sport" (2016) 9 (6) Origins *Current Events in Historical Perspective*
21 John Hobberman, *Mortal Engines-the Science of Performance and the Dehumanization of Sport* (The Blackburn Press, 1992)
22 Ibid 6

regard to the betting industry, primarily horse racing.[23] The spread of antipathy for PEDs from horse racing to human sports thus needs to be contextualized. The rise of the IOC and its stance on the questions of amateurism versus professionalism set the tone of the subsequent policy on PEDs.

Ahoy amateurism! Gimmick or concern of the IOC?

The IOC began its journey by propagating the idea of amateurism. Baron Pierre de Coubertin, the father of the modern Olympics, was keen on portraying sports as honest and morally pure.[24] The IOC coined a smart catchphrase viz. amateurism. It gradually developed and gained momentum as the years passed.[25] Coubertin's noble intentions of promoting not-for-profit sport enabled the IOC to increase its commercial value. Amateurism was used as a smart marketing tool to initially establish Olympic sports as an elite and exclusive group of activity.[26] It distinguished the ethos of working class from nobility.[27] Thus the Olympic brand was created, symbolizing a puritan form of activity called "Olympic sport." Consequently, all the sports federations seeking IOC recognition had to strictly follow the principles of amateurism.[28]

The IAAF, as mentioned above, became the first International Sports Federation (ISF) to uphold the principles of amateurism. Its founder and chairman, J. Sigfrid Edstrom, was a staunch proponent of amateurism. He exemplifies the reasons that facilitated the spread of PED antipathy from animal sports to human sports. He ensured that the IAAF maintained the strict divide between amateurism and professionalism. Accordingly, in 1928 Edstrom got the IAAF to adopt a formal definition of doping. As per this definition, use of PEDs (specifically stimulants) to increase athletic skills beyond average was doping. Along with the definition, the IAAF also specified sanctions to be imposed in the event of doping rule violation,[29] which in most cases involved suspension from all forms

23 Charles E. Yesalis and Michael S. Bahrke (n 16) 47
24 Dikaia Chatziefstathiou, "The Changing Nature of the Ideology of Olympism in the Modern Olympic Era" https://dspace.lboro.ac.uk/dspace-jspui/bitstream/2134/2820/1/THESIS_FINAL%20090605_sb.pdf (accessed 23 June 2018)
25 Christoph Bertling, "The Loss of Profit? The Rise of Professionalism in the Olympic Movement and the Consequences for National Sport Systems" (2007) 2 *Journal of Olympic History* 50 http://library.la84.org/SportsLibrary/JOH/JOHv15n2/JOHv15n2m.pdf (accessed 23 June 2018)
26 Rob Beamish, *Steroids: A New Look at Performance Enhancing Drugs* (Praeger, 2011)
27 Mark Johnson (n 15) 35–36
28 Matthew P. Llewellyn and John Gleaves, "The Rise of the Shamateur The International Olympic Committee, Broken-Time Payments, and the Preservation of the Amateur Ideal, 1925–1930" (2014) XXIII *Olympika* 1 http://library.la84.org/SportsLibrary/Olympika/Olympika_2014/olympika2014c.pdf (25 June 2018)
29 For details See Handbook of the International Amateur Athletic Federation-1927–28 www.iaaf.org/download/download?filename=bd61cf34-14b2-4dfc-9745-de91; www.iaaf.org/news/news/a-piece-of-anti-doping-history-iaaf-handbook (accessed 24October 2018)

of amateur athletics. The justification of this first notable anti-doping rule clearly resides in the concept of amateurism. Edstrom was also a prominent member of the IOC, serving as vice president and later president between 1946 and 1952. Hence, he carried his views on amateurism to the policy-making process within the IOC.[30] Thus, amateurism became the major catalyst and reason for the gradual development of anti-doping policies within the IOC framework. Amateurism was treated as a sacrosanct principle, and preservation of the same was the stated mission of the IOC.[31]

Understandably, the preservation of this holier-than-thou attitude of the IOC needed strictures against all practices contrary to the idea of amateurism. The IOC Charter of 1933, for instance, outlines the virtues of an amateur by insisting that a "true sportsman" is the one who plays sports for the sake of it without any other motive. The pure joy of participation was eulogized. Monetary gain was derided and looked down upon. Olympism was referred to as the epitome of moral purity and nobility.[32] Losing, as opposed to winning by use of unfair means, was vehemently discouraged. The 1938 Charter champions the cause of amateurism further, by introducing stringent consequences for fraudulently misrepresenting oneself as an amateur. An athlete who was found to be misrepresenting their status was to be disqualified and lose all winnings.[33] In essence the words "professionalism" and "commercialism" were taboo for the IOC. In hindsight this was the smartest move the IOC could have come up with to earn revenue.

The ideology of amateurism was in contrast to the political realities of the period.[34] Nonetheless, Coubertin insisted on it to please the anglophiles and elites of the West.[35] The lack of sincerity in the IOC's belief in amateurism is evident from the fact that the IOC Charters did not define the concept.[36] It

30 Leif Yttergren, "J. Sigfrid Edstrom and the Nurmi Affair of 1932: The Struggle of the Amateur Fundamentalists Against Professionalism in the Olympic Movement" (2007) 15 (3) *Journal of Olympic History* 21 library.la84.org/SportsLibrary/JOH/JOHv15n3/JOHv15n3h.pdf (accessed 24 October 2018)

31 Ian Ritchie, "Understanding Performance Enhancing Substances and Sanctions Against their Use from the Perspective of History" in Verner Moller, Ivan Waddington and John M. Hobberman (eds.), *Routledge Handbook of Drugs and Sport* (Routledge, 2015)

32 Olympic Charter, 1933 https://stillmed.olympic.org/media/Document%20Library/OlympicOrg/ Olympic-Studies-Centre/List-of-Resources/Official-Publications/Olympic-Charters/EN-1933- Olympic-Charter.pdf#_ga=2.39123050.833335678.1529663796-130387347.1524895071 (accessed 23 June 2018)

33 Olympic Charter, 1938, Rule 17 https://stillmed.olympic.org/media/Document%20Library/ OlympicOrg/Olympic-Studies-Centre/List-of-Resources/Official-Publications/Olympic-Charters/ EN-1938-Olympic-Charter-Olympic-Rules.pdf#_ga=2.140216692.692104528.1529993269- 130387347.1524895071 (accessed 25 June 2018)

34 Matthew P. Llewellyn and John Gleaves (n 28)

35 Ibid 4–5

36 In the Olympic Charter 1930, for instance, the part dealing with the definition *amateur* reads as "The definition of an amateur as drawn up by the respective International Federations of Sport is recognized for the admission of athletes taking part in the Olympic Games. Where

left that task to individual federations. Additionally, the IOC also delegated responsibility for enforcing the rule of amateurism entirely to the International Federations.[37] This delegation enabled the IOC to maintain an ambiguous stance on the regulation of amateurism.[38] It further provided flexibility to the IOC to seek corporate sponsorship for the Olympic Games, while prohibiting the same for the athletes. Visible change was evidenced in the 1928 Olympic Games, where the organizers went for a sponsorship with Coca-Cola.[39] While there were protestations within the IOC, it did not reverse the trend. Soon the Olympic motto and symbols were commodified. Gradually, the IOC became completely involved in the marketing and commercial exploitation of the Olympic Games.[40]

The duality of the IOC's approach definitely affected the enforcement of amateurism within Olympic sports.[41] Strict compliance with the principle of amateurism was never put into practice by the IOC. A glaring example of the IOC's ambivalent attitude towards amateurism can be gleaned from the IOC's Executive Committee meeting of August 1927. In this meeting, held in Paris, the IOC Executive Committee resolved to provide monetary compensation to the International Federation of the Football Association (FIFA). This was a measure aimed at compensating football players' lost earnings and incentivizing their participation in the Olympics.[42] Understandably then, the IOC Charters since 1908 had no official response to the use of PEDs in Olympic sports. Doping is mentioned for the first time in the IOC Charter of 1946. Considering that by 1928 the Olympic Games had been commercialized, the hardening stance on PEDs appears only as a public relation exercise. The ineffectiveness of this stance is evident from the fact that post-1946 there were allegations of

---

there is no International Federation governing a sport, the definition shall be drawn up by the Organizing Committee, in agreement with the I.0. C. The National Association, which in each country governs each particular sport, must certify on the special form that each competitor is an amateur in accordance with the rules of the International Federation governing that sport." https://stillmed.olympic.org/media/Document%20Library/OlympicOrg/Olympic-Studies-Centre/List-of-Resources/Official-Publications/Olympic-Charters/EN-1930-Olympic Charter.pdf#_ga=2.191807785.2044814159.1530516709-130387347.1524895071 (accessed 2 July 2019)

37 Ibid 24

38 Matthew P. Llewellyn and John Gleaves (n 28) 5

39 Rob Beamish and Ian Ritchie, *Fastest, Highest, Strongest-a Critique of High-performance Sports* (Routledge, 2006)

40 Robert K. Barney, "An Olympian Dilemma: Protection of Olympic Symbols" (2002) 10 (3) *Journal of Olympic History* 7–9 http://library.la84.org/SportsLibrary/JOH/JOHv10n3/JOHv10n3f.pdf (accessed 2 July 2018)

41 Matthew P. Llewellyn and John T. Gleaves, "The Rise of the 'Shamateur' The International Olympic Committee and the Preservation of the Amateur Idea" http://library.la84.org/Sports-Library/ISOR/isor2012h.pdf (accessed 3 July 2018)

42 Official Bulletin of the International Olympic Committee, "Minutes of the Meeting of the Executive Committee Paris 8th August 1927" http://library.la84.org/OlympicInformationCenter/OlympicReview/1927/BODE8/BODE8g.pdf (accessed 3 July 2018)

doping by athletes participating in the 1948 Olympics.[43] Thus PEDs were never strictly regulated by the IOC. As is evident from the 1946 Charter, doping was only condemned and not prohibited or declared illegal. Ironically, the IOC stood by as amateurs continued using performance enhancers, following in the footsteps of the professionals.[44] Only when the IOC's public image suffered a beating did it come out with an anti-doping policy. Maintaining a clean public image was needed to legitimize the ideology of amateurism. The scandals that rocked the sporting world were used not to acknowledge the flaws in the system, but rather as another reason to buttress the public stance on amateurism and purity of sport.

Scandals and the IOC: scripting the anti-doping narrative

The IOC used Knud Enemark Jensen's death at the 1960 Rome Olympics to turn the tide against the use of PEDs. Since then, the IOC has continuously developed an anti-doping narrative that suits its agenda. The IOC used Jensen's death to justify its anti-doping policy that was officially brought to force following the 1960 Olympics. However, circumstantial evidence, culled from various sources, reveals a different picture of the cause of Jensen's death. Jensen was reported to have taken Roniacol which is meant to dilate the blood vessels, ensuring a greater supply of blood. However, one of its possible side effects is dizziness leading to fainting. Hence, Roniacol appears to be less than conducive to enhancing performance. Another important factor was the hot Italian weather. On the day of the race the weather was extremely hot. The team of Danish bicycle riders, of which Jensen was a member, was struggling against the heat.[45]

At the start of the race the Danes had four team members, but soon one of them suffered from heatstroke and had to be rushed to the hospital. Since Olympic rules required a minimum of three riders to complete the race or else face the threat of disqualification, Jensen and his two teammates had to finish the race. Five kilometres before the finish line Jensen was in serious discomfort. He was struggling to such an extent that his two teammates had to hold his shirt, thus keeping him from slipping. Soon though Jensen completely lost his grip and slipped from the cycle, his head hitting the road. Jensen was overwhelmed by heatstroke. Things worsened further when the ambulance rushed him to a tent which was even warmer. The situation turned dire, and Jensen

---

43 John Gleaves, "Doped Professionals and Clean Amateurs: Amateurism's Influence on the Modern Philosophy of Anti-Doping" (2011) 38 (2) *Journal of Sport History* 248
44 Mark Johnson (n 15) 60–61
45 Peter Christensen, "The Drama About the Olympics in Rome" *Politiken* (2008) https://politiken.dk/kultur/boger/faglitteratur_boger/art4779455/Dramaet-om-OL-i-Rom (accessed 7 July 2018)

died inside the tent.[46] The autopsy noted that Jensen died because of heat-stroke and not due to PED use.[47] Unfortunately, the subsequent discussions and debates on the causes of Jensen's death have been simplified to an open-and-shut case of doping-related death. His death is used to exemplify the vices of PEDs and to instill fear in the minds of athletes.[48] His death was used by the IOC to lay the foundation of a medical commission to investigate the issue of doping in the Olympics.

The media was fed the news that Jensen died due to doping, and the IOC latched onto the negative publicity to justify its subsequent anti-doping measures.[49] The stance of the IOC thus drastically changed. Earlier the IOC had been circumspect about the dangers of PEDs to the ethos of amateurism. Anti-doping thus was a subset principle of amateurism. Post-Jensen, the IOC adopted anti-doping as a concept paralleling and equal to the stature of amateurism. Subsequently, anti-doping took on the stature of a moral principle that eventually overshadowed amateurism. The overhyping of anti-doping was fostered by men who portrayed doping as inherently immoral irrespective of its impact on an athlete. The first of these men was Avery Brundage, a close associate of Sigfrid Edstrom. As discussed above, Edstrom was a staunch supporter of amateurism. Brundage was clearly inspired, for he, too, was an amateurism fundamentalist.[50] Brundage's obsession with amateurism was fanatical. His obduracy with amateurism led the IOC to revise the Olympic Oath in 1956 under which an athlete was to promise to remain an amateur for life.[51] Brundage therefore used this obsession to build up a strong anti-doping regime. And in this he was supported by another sports moralist, Antonio Venerando, who firmly believed that doping was sports fraud. Hence, ethical sports required stringent anti-doping measures.[52]

46 Peter Christensen (n 45) A photo in the Danish newspaper Extra Bladet shows Jensen's shirt being held by his two mates https://journalisten.dk/billeder/fotograf/ekstra-bladets-fotograf-busser-fotograferede-under-ol-i-rom-i-1960-den-dopede-cyke (accessed 7 July 2018)
47 Paul Dimeo, "The Truth About Knud: Revisiting an Anti-Doping Myth" *Sports Integrity Initiative* sportsintegrityinitiative.com (accessed 25 October 2018)
48 Verner Møller, "Knud Enemark Jensen's Death During the 1960 Rome Olympics: A Search for Truth?" (2005) 25 (3) *Sport in History* 452 www.academia.dk/Blog/wp-content/uploads/VernerMoller_KnudEnemark.pdf (accessed 7 July 2018)
49 Aaron Gordon, "The Morality Myth Behind the Modern Anti-Doping Movement" (2017) Vice Sports sports.vice.com (accessed 27 October 2018)
50 Maynard Brichford, "Avery Brundage on Amateurism: Preaching and Practice" http://library.la84.org/SportsLibrary/ISOR/isor2010k.pdf (accessed 29 October 2018)
51 James Murray, "Olympians Put Avery Brundage on The Spot" *Sports Illustrated Vault* (1956) www.si.com/vault/1956/08/27/584401/olympians-put-avery-brundage-on-the-spot (accessed 30 October 2018)
52 Paul Dimeo, "The Myth of Clean Sport and Its Unintended Consequences" (2016) 4 (3–4) *Performance Enhancement and Health* 103 https://dspace.stir.ac.uk/bitstream/1893/23155/1/The%20Myth%20of%20Clean%20Sport%20%28with%20corrections%29%20updated.pdf (accessed 1 November 2018)

The most influential member of this think tank was Prof Ludwig Prokop, who was one of the strongest critics of doping in sports from the 1950s.[53] He was against doping primarily because doping, as per his view, was unfair and against principles of equal competition.[54] For him, anti-doping measures were needed to preserve the purity of sport.[55] These men thus ensured that the IOC would enthusiastically focus on doping in sports. Others chimed in to the growing chorus calling for the adoption of full-fledged anti-doping measures, including dope tests. For instance, at the Moscow International Olympic Committee Session held in June 1962, members urged the IOC to test urine samples, impose a penalty for doping and to conduct an anti-doping awareness programme.[56] This demand mirrored the same concern expressed by Brundage, Ludwig et al. viz. that doping is an evil that is out to destroy sports. The anti-doping narrative thus was transformed into a debate between good versus evil, where use of PEDs was portrayed as inherently evil. This narrative was formalized and codified with the establishment of the IOC Medical Commission,[57] whose first head was Sir Arthur Porritt, a doctor by profession.[58] Sir Porritt had similar views as those of Avery Brundage. According to Sir Porritt, doping per se was amoral and personified evil itself.[59] This was significant, because the IOC Medical Commission was tasked with crafting the anti-doping roadmap. Although the IOC Medical Commission did not achieve anything significant under the leadership of Sir Porritt,[60] he nevertheless prompted debates on drug testing and sanctions against athletes testing positive for doping. He proposed that testing

53 Ludwig Prokop, "Drug Abuse in International Athletics" (1975) 3 (2) Journal of Sports Medicine 85

54 Gazetta, "Doping" in Ludwig Prokop (ed.), Success in Sport – Theory and Practice of Performance Enhancement (1) www.cycling4fans.de/index.php?id=5302 (accessed 2 November 2018). Also see Ludwig Prokop, "The Contribution of Sports Medicine to the Improvement of Performances" 46 http://library.la84.org/OlympicInformationCenter/OlympicReview/1978/ore123/ore123l.pdf (accessed 2 November 2018)

55 Paul Dimeo, A History of Drug Use in Sports-1876–1976-beyond Good and Evil (Routledge, 2007)

56 Report and Restatement of the Question of Doping, Presented at the Moscow International Olympic Committee Session in June 1962 by Dr J. Ferreira Santos titled "Doping" http://library. la84.org/OlympicInformationCenter/OlympicReview/1963/BDCE81/BDCE81u.pdf (accessed 2 November 2018)

57 Ian Ritchie, "Before and After 1968: Reconsidering the Introduction of Drug Testing in the Olympic Games" in Stephen Wagg (ed.), Myths and Milestones in the History of Sport (Palgrave Macmillan, 2011)

58 For more information on Sir Arthur Porritt see www.olympic.org.nz/athletes/arthur-porritt/ (accessed 8 November 2018)

59 Rob Beamish, "Chapter VII. Olympic Ideals versus the Performance Imperative: The History of Canada's Anti-Doping Policies" in Lucie Thibault and Jean Harvey (ed.), Sport Policy in Canada (University of Ottawa Press, 2013) https://books.openedition.org/uop/711?lang=en (accessed 8 November 2018)

60 International Olympic Committee, "Medical Commission-overview of the Content of the Archives Concerning the History, Missions and Activities of the IOC Medical Commission from 1936 to 1995" https://stillmed.olympic.org/media/Document%20Library/

should be outsourced and that the Olympic Organizing Committee should only play a supervisory role.[61] These debates thus focused not on the viability of banning drugs but on the severity of punishment and the extent of testing. Sir Porritt proposed that even organizations proven to be involved in doping should be sanctioned.[62]

The narrative of good versus evil did not stem the craze for PEDs. A glaring example of this was the death of Tom Simpson on 13 July 1967 during the Tour de France. His autopsy revealed the use of amphetamines, a widely used PED.[63] This was both a reflection of the flawed IOC policy of banning PEDs as well professional sports taking over amateur sports. Nonetheless, the IOC, along with the other International Sports Federations, continued to devise a more stringent anti-doping policy. Sir Porritt stepped down in 1967 and was succeeded by Prince Alexandre de Merode.[64] As mentioned above, Sir Porritt's leadership was slow to define a clear-cut policy on doping.[65] Only in 1967 do we find concrete proposals being put forth in the 65th Session of the IOC to tackle doping.[66] The minutes of this session note the modalities to be put in place for dope testing, as well as documenting the list of prohibited substances.[67] This was a new beginning for the IOC Medical Commission under the leadership of Prince Merode. Under his leadership drug testing was done for the first time during the 1968 Olympic Games.[68] However, de Merode was a political figure, and lacked any scientific knowledge, which probably explains how he managed to be at the helm of the IOC Medical Commission from 1967 to 2002, the year he died.[69] Nonetheless he

OlympicOrg/Olympic-Studies-Centre/List-of-Resources/Resources-available/Archives/EN-Medical-Commission.pdf (accessed 8 November 2018)

61 Avery Brundage, "The IOC and Medical Problems" http://library.la84.org/OlympicInformation Center/OlympicReview/1968/ore11/ore11f.pdf (accessed 8 November 2018)

62 Michael Kremenik, Sho Onodera, Mitsushiro Nagao, Osamu Yuzuki and Shozo Yonetani, "A Historical Timeline of Doping in the Olympics (Part 1 1896–1968)" (2006) 12 (1) *Kawasaki Journal of Medical Welfare* 19 www.kawasaki-m.ac.jp/soc/mw/journal/en/2006-e12-1/01_kremenik.pdf (accessed 8 November 2018)

63 Patrick Mignon, "The Tour de France and the Doping Issue" (2003) 20 (2) *International Journal of the History of Sport*, Taylor Francis (Routledge) 227 https://hal-insep.archives-ouvertes.fr/hal-01697488/document (accessed 8 November 2018)

64 Arne Ljungqvist, "Brief History of Anti-Doping" in O Rabin and Y Pitsiladis (eds.), *Acute Topics in Anti-Doping. Medicine and Sport Science* 62 (Basel, Karger, 2017) www.karger.com/WebMaterial/ShowFileCache/877472 (accessed 9 November 2018)

65 Ibid

66 See "Extracts of the minutes of the 65th session of the International Olympic Committee Tehran, 6, 7, and 8 May 1967" http://library.la84.org/OlympicInformationCenter/OlympicReview/1967/BDCE98/BDCE98w.pdf (accessed 10 November 2018)

67 Ibid

68 Paul Dimeo and Thomas Hunt, "Leading Anti-Doping in the IOC-the Ambiguous Role of Prince Alexandre de Merode" (2009) 17 (1) *Journal of Olympic History* 20 http://library.la84.org/Sports Library/JOH/JOHv17n1/JOHv17n1g.pdf (accessed 13 November 2018)

69 Obituaries, "Prince Alexandre de Mrode" *The Telegraph* (London, 27 November 2002) www.telegraph.co.uk/news/obituaries/1414375/Prince-Alexandre-de-Merode.html (accessed 13 November 2018)

was an anti-doping hardliner, firmly believing that doping is against the morality of sport. In addition, the IOC Medical Commission of 1967 included figures such as Prof Prokop, who was also a doping hardliner. Thus, from the beginning the IOC Medical Commission's agenda was to develop anti-doping policies premised primarily on the principles of morality.[70]

The Ben Johnson episode: testing times for the IOC?

The zero-tolerance anti-doping policy could not ebb the use of drugs in sports. On the contrary, the doping scandals were getting bigger and better. One of the most talked about and discussed doping scandals involved track and field athlete Ben Johnson. On 24 September 1988, Johnson became the fastest man on earth, setting a world record of 9.79 seconds. Canada was ecstatic, and so was the world. Johnson had ended the domination of the US in athletics, and everyone was celebrating the new Olympic Champion.[71] The race was, at that point in time, touted as the greatest race in the history of sports. Understandably, when the news of Johnson having doped broke out, it was the biggest scandal to hit sports at that point in time.[72] He tested positive for the anabolic steroid stanozolol and was stripped of his gold medal and world record.[73] Canada reacted swiftly and constituted the Dubin Commission of Inquiry, headed by Charles L. Dubin. The committee met in October 1988 and submitted its report in 1990.[74] A perusal

70 Kathryn E Henne, "The Origins of the International Olympic Committee Medical Commission and Its Technocratic Regime: An Historiographic Investigation of Anti-Doping Regulation and Enforcement in International Sport" www.academia.edu/530687/The_Origins_of_the_Interna tional_Olympic_Committee_Medical_Commission_and_its_Technocratic_Regime_An_Histo riographic_Investigation_of_Anti-Doping_ (accessed 15 November 2018)

71 Andrea Mann, "September 27, 1988: Ben Johnson Is Stripped of His Olympic Gold Medal After Failing Drugs Test the Most Famous Men's 100m Final in the History of the Olympics Became the Most Infamous When Canadian Sprinter Ben Johnson Was Found Guilty of Taking Steroids" BT (Montreal, 26 September 2018) http://home.bt.com/news/on-this-day/september-27-1988-ben-johnson-is-stripped-of-his-olympic-gold-medal-after-failing-drugs-test-11364007354384 (accessed 16 November 2018)

72 Jack Moore, "Throwback Thursday: Ben Johnson at the Seoul Olympics, and the Doping Race That Never Ends Ben Johnson's 100m Dash Victory and Subsequent Steroid Bust at the 1988 Summer Games Was a Watershed Moment for Anti-Doping activists, but to what end?" Vice Sports (Montreal, 24 September 2015) https://sports.vice.com/en_ca/article/53v7xd/throwback-thursday-ben-johnson-at-the-seoul-olympics-and-the-doping-race-that-never-ends (accessed 16 November 2018)

73 Patrick Maloney, "Ben Johnson scandal 25 Years Later" Ottawa Sun (Ottawa, 22 September 2013) https://ottawasun.com/2013/09/22/ben-johnson-scandal-25-years-later/wcm/7a445688-6861-40b3-a21f-665404f11699 (accessed 16 November 2018)

74 The Honourable Charles L. Dubin Commissioner, Commission of Inquiry into the Use of Drugs and Banned Practices Intended to Increase Athletic Performance (Canadian Government Publishing Centre, 1990) www.doping.nl/media/kb/3636/Dubin-report-1990-eng%20(S).pdf (accessed 16 November 2018)

of the report brings out the gaping flaw in the anti-doping policy propagated by the IOC and its members. The report reveals an organized doping programme being carried out by Johnson with the help of his team. It was done with the full consent of Johnson in a sophisticated manner with utmost secrecy. Interestingly, people associated with the doping programme were all accredited and authorized by the Canadian National Olympic Committee to train Johnson.[75] And they duped the Canadian National Olympic Committee by conducting the surreptitious anti-doping programme.

The evidence, as provided in the Dubin report, proves that officials in the highest positions of sports governance turned a blind eye to the organized doping programme.[76] Even the Canadian Track and Field Association (CTFA) appeared to implicitly encourage the doping programme.[77] The 1988 Olympic sprint team from Canada was composed of coaches, doctors and a therapist rumored to run the doping programme.[78] Johnson, on being questioned by the committee, admitted to the use of PEDs. He conceded to being aware of all the anti-doping rules, including the consequences upon being caught. Johnson was equally encouraged by the inherent failure of the dope testing systems. He was, as noted in the Dubin report, tested nineteen times from 1986 up to 1988. He never tested positive, and thus was never caught prior to the Seoul Olympics.[79] Hence, at the Seoul Olympics, Johnson and the Canadian Olympic sprint team were confident that all would be smooth sailing. However, the doping plan for Seoul misfired, as the administration of the PEDs did not go according to plan. As the Dubin report details, the execution of the last doping scheme was done within a time frame very close to the 100 m event. Consequently, the traces of PEDs given to Johnson could not be washed out from his system and he was caught.[80]

The Johnson episode should have acted as a wake-up call for the IOC and its member federations. As mentioned above, there was a failure to investigate the allegations pertaining to Johnson's training programme. The failure was of the Canadian sports agencies who were deputed by the IOC and IAAF to govern the sports and stringently follow the anti-doping programme.[81] Further, Johnson was willing to be part of the doping programme, hence forgoing the principles of amateurism. He, like any other professional, was seeking help to improve his performance. His coach, doctor and therapist were providing him that help. There is no documentation that Johnson developed any serious health issues as a result of the doping programme. It was consensual and without coercion. The

---

75 Ibid 201
76 Ibid 202–213
77 Charles L. Dubin (n 74) 225
78 Ibid 234–235
79 Ibid 285
80 Ibid 300
81 For information on organizational structure of IOC see "The Organisation" www.olympic.org/about-ioc-institution (accessed 18 November 2018)

IOC and IAAF should have hauled up their agents for the transgressions. They should have re-examined their stated position against doping. Instead, doping was reinforced as a case of deviance and subject of contempt. IOC president Juan Antonio Samaranch admitted that the whole incident was a setback to the Olympic movement. At the same time, Samaranch insisted that the successful detection of doping legitimized the IOC's strict anti-doping stance.[82] The Dubin report, however, undermined Samaranch's stance, stating that the use of PEDs was widely prevalent across all countries and in almost all sports. The report cited two main reasons for the failure of the existing anti-doping programme. The first was that the use of PEDs was being done secretly, and the second was that the officials in charge of carrying out the anti-doping programme failed in the discharge of their duties.[83]

The IOC's incompetency is further evidenced by the fact that the extensive inquiry into the doping scandal of 1988 was initiated by the Canadian government. Neither the IOC nor the IAAF had any role to play in the investigations that were conducted. This indicates a lack of will on the part of the governing bodies and the IOC to acknowledge flaws within the anti-doping narrative. The most telling statement in the Dubin report is on page 350, where it is stated that the inquiry led to the discovery of widespread doping across board. And this is regarded as a global disgrace.[84] In addition, the significance of the statement also lies in the fact that this discovery was done notwithstanding the existing anti-doping measures. As per the Dubin report, the failure of the anti-doping programme was due to several reasons. The first was the ease of access to the banned substances, facilitated by the widespread manufacture, importation and distribution of the same.[85] Understandably, the IOC was not in a position to check these sources. It needed the state to do so. Second, though not identified as such, most of the drugs banned by the IOC had legitimate medical uses. Accordingly, their manufacture could not be completely stopped. The most the Dubin report hoped for was stricter regulation.[86] This brings forth the most interesting aspect of the anti-doping programme, for the entire premise of banning drugs in sports is proven to be not based on health concerns at all. The moralistic premise of spirit of sport and unfairness gets highlighted as the credo. Unfortunately, the Dubin report neither acknowledges nor discusses this problem in the anti-doping ideology. On the contrary, doping is sought to be eliminated through stricter rules, to be framed by the state.

82 Christine Brennan, "IOC Strips Johnson of Gold Medal in 100" *The Washington Post* (Washington, 27 September 1988) www.washingtonpost.com/archive/politics/1988/09/27/ioc-strips-johnson-of-gold-medal-in-100/9cd59877-87c4-44ec-9e96-69eb58f37fa2/?utm_term=.6c35b78036b1 (accessed 18 November 2018)

83 Charles L. Dubin (n 74) 335–336

84 Ibid 350

85 Ibid 369

86 Ibid 378

The other problems identified by the Dubin report pertained to flaws in the testing programme of the IOC viz. only in-competition testing and conflict of interest in the accreditation of laboratories.[87] The Dubin report reaffirms the moralist stand vis-à-vis sports and derides both commercialization and professionalization of sports. Accordingly, the recommendations were premised on this moral and ethical aspect of sport.[88] Such an approach would not help in dealing with the doping problem, because it does not acknowledge the professionalization of sports as an irreversible reality. Interestingly, the recommendation does not dismiss the requirement of achieving excellence in elite sports, understandably so because no recommendation would be acceptable if it did not highlight the importance of excelling in sports. In real terms, this also means winning medals and adding to the glory of the nation. And glorification of winning in sports would inevitably incentivize the use of PEDs. One measure that the Dubin report recommended to deal with doping was for the effective coordination between the state and the sports governing bodies. This creates scope for enforcing accountability within the sports governing bodies and acts as a check against exploitation or discrimination by sports governing bodies.[89] The other significant recommendation of the Dubin report was to introduce out-of-competition testing,[90] and a transparent tendering procedure was recommended as a viable method ensure the accuracy of the laboratories and to avoid conflict-of-interest scenarios.[91] Overall the recommendations were far-reaching and well-intentioned, but, as stated above, they were not enough. The Johnson saga was not the last of the doping-related controversies, nor was the IOC's anti-doping programme safe from further attacks.

The Festina affair – the end of the road for the IOC Medical Commission?

The next big shocker was the Festina affair, which threatened the survival of the Tour de France and impacted the world of sports like never before. On 8 July 1998, French customs officials seized a car full of PEDs. The car belonged to Willy Voet, a Belgian physiotherapist and member of the Festina team. One thing led to another, and the French authorities conducted a series of raids and arrests for trafficking and possession of PEDs.[92] This incident changed the narrative of the anti-doping programme by criminalizing the possession and use of PEDs. Earlier the use of PEDs had essentially been a sports affair, confined to the

87 Ibid 394–411
88 Ibid 515–517
89 Ibid 530
90 Ibid 541–542
91 Ibid 542–543
92 Detlef Hacke, "From Festina to Team Telekom/Team T-Mobile – Doping Scandals in Cycling" www.uni-freiburg.de/universitaet/einzelgutachten/symposium-freiburg-2011-hacke.pdf (accessed 21 November 2018)

jurisdiction of the IOC and the sport governing bodies. With Festina, it changed into an affair of the state. The incident exposed the incompetency of the IOC Medical Commission and other anti-doping organizations.[93] Juan Antonio Samaranch, the IOC president during the Festina affair, was embattled. As mentioned earlier, after Johnson, Festina rocked his presidency. In between there were allegations that Samaranch was instrumental in covering up several cases of doping.[94] Post Festina, Samaranch was also attacked for heading one of the most corrupt periods of the IOC.[95]

The IOC was faced with an existential crisis, and Samaranch, with the help of de Merode, went into PR mode. They were desperate to ward-off direct interference from the state. The threat from the state was personified by the acts of the French government. Tough measures followed suit, with the French government passing laws criminalizing the use of PEDs in sports.[96] The challenge to the IOC's credibility threatened the organization's lucrative corporate sponsorships. Hence, as in the past, the whole anti-doping policy façade needed to be repaired and restored in order to ensure the commercial sustainability of the IOC.[97] Samaranch convened a world conference on doping in sport scheduled from 2–4 February 1999 in Lausanne, Switzerland.[98] The plan was to assert the superiority and legitimacy of the IOC vis-à-vis the anti-doping policy formulation. However, Samaranch and de Merode's vacillations over enforcement of anti-doping measures and denial of failures weakened the IOC's stand.[99] The agenda was also to replace the IOC Medical Commission with an IOC-controlled doping agency. The IOC had decided upon the name of the agency viz. Olympic Movement Anti-Doping Agency.[100]

93 Sarah Teetzel, ""The Road to WADA" Cultural Relations Old and New: The Transitory Olympic Ethos" (2004) Seventh International Symposium for Olympic Research 213 https://digital.la84. org/digital/collection/p17103coll10/id/13553/rec/4 (accessed 22 November 2018)

94 Duncan Mackay, "Samaranch to Lead Drug Agency" The Guardian (London, 2 February 1999) www.theguardian.com/sport/1999/feb/02/samaranch-head-anti-doping-agency (accessed 22 November 2018)

95 Obituary, "Marc Hodler: Exposed Scandal in Selection of Olympics' Host Cities" Associated Press (Lausanne, 20 October 2006) www.washingtonpost.com/wp-dyn/content/article/2006/10/19/AR2006101901725.html (accessed 22 November 2018)

96 "World: Europe French doping crackdown" BBC (London, 19 November 1998) http://news.bbc.co.uk/2/hi/europe/217845.stm (accessed 23 November 2018)

97 John Hoberman, Testosterone Dreams: Rejuvenation, Aphrodisia, Doping (University of California Press, 2005)

98 Dag Vidar Hanstad, Andy Smith and Ivan Waddington, "The Establishment of the World Anti-Doping Agency: A Study of the Management of Organizational Change and Unplanned Outcomes" www.researchgate.net/profile/Ivan_Waddington/publication/233540368_The_Establishment_of_the_World_Anti-Doping_Agency_A_Study_of_the_Management_of_Organizational_Change_and_Unplanned_Outcomes/links/55ad1b7008aee079921d510e/The-Establishment-of-the-World-Anti-Doping-Agency-A-Study-of-the-Management-of-Organizational-Change-and-Unplanned-Outcomes.pdf (accessed 23 November 2018)

99 Ibid 7

100 Ibid 15

In short, the Lausanne Conference was convened to attempt preempting the Western countries who were furious with the spate of scandals.[101] Understandably so, because countries like the US, UK, France *et al.* had been supportive of the spirit of sport narrative and the IOC's philosophy on doping. Hence, they could visualize the fall of this ideology due to the IOC's incompetency.[102] De Merode did not help matters, because as the head of the IOC Medical Commission he had gone on record in support of a flexible sanction regime. The laxity of Samaranch and his men was evident.[103] Post-Festina, the consensus amongst Western countries was to strengthen the anti-doping measures, and thus the conference was an apt platform. The representatives of the leading sports powers, like the US, UK and France, vented their pent-up anger against the IOC's inaction.[104] As a result, the IOC's plan to have complete control over anti-doping policies and implementation failed. The outcome was not an IOC-controlled doping agency but an independent anti-doping agency, outside the control of the IOC, funded by both governments as well as the IOC.[105] The Lausanne Declaration on Doping in Sport was adopted on 4 February 1999, which set forth the creation of the International Anti-Doping Agency.[106] The declaration reflected the sentiments of a wide group of stakeholders viz. governments as well non-governmental organizations. Thus, it was not confined to the IOC and its members, as originally planned.

The Lausanne Declaration rejected the IOC's stance on various issues, including sanctions. Thus, the declaration set forth a uniform sanction of two years. It recognized the importance of both in-competition and out-of-competition testing. Importantly, the declaration emphasized the importance of coordination between the sports governing bodies and the governmental organizations.[107] This was a realization which was now documented in the post-Festina realities. The declaration therefore was a death knell to the existence of the IOC Medical Commission. The new anti-doping agency was expected to be operationalized during the 2000 Summer Olympics at Sydney, Australia. The journey of the IOC Medical Commission was cut short, highlighting that the IOC clearly failed in its commitments. Interestingly, despite all of this, neither the IOC nor its members

101 Ibid 14
102 John Hoberman, "Backtalk: Offering the Illusion of Reform on Drugs" *The New York Times* (New York, 10 January 1999)
103 Jere Longman, "Olympics: I.O.C. Drug Chief Calls for Shift in Bans" *The New York Times* (New York, 29 January 1999)
104 Philip Hersh, "IOC Anti-Doping 'Declaration' Is No Victory for Samaranch" *Chicago Tribune* (Chicago, 5 February 1999) www.chicagotribune.com/news/ct-xpm-1999-02-05-9902050084-story.html (accessed 23 November 2018)
105 Dag Vidar Hanstad, Andy Smith and Ivan Waddington (n 98) 19
106 "Lausanne Declaration on Doping in Sport-adopted by the World Conference on Doping in Sport 4 February 1999, Lausanne, Switzerland" www.wada-ama.org/sites/default/files/resources/files/lausanne_declaration_on_doping_in_sport.pdf (accessed 24 November 2018)
107 Ibid

such as the IAAF, Union Cycliste Internationale (UCI) *et al.* were completely barred from carrying out anti-doping measures. Further, the governments to play a major role in structuring the new agency were all from developed, First World countries. Finally, the concerns of the athletes that were mentioned in the declaration were again those of the elite First World athlete. The important issue was that there were no reflections of any larger concerns. This was understandable because the declaration was reactionary in nature, with the aim of preventing the occurrence of another Festina-like affair.

WADA and the Convention – legitimization within!

The Lausanne Declaration led to the establishment of the World Anti-Doping Agency (WADA) on 10 November 1999.[108] As the name indicates, this was clearly a departure from the IOC's original plan of controlling the anti-doping programme.[109] The governments were serious about having a major say in anti-doping regulation.[110] One of the significant steps taken to distance WADA from the IOC was the selection of Montreal as the headquarters of WADA.[111] Originally, WADA was headquartered in Lausanne. However, because the IOC was headquartered in Lausanne, WADA's head office was shifted to Montreal in 2002.[112] The next step was to ensure equal participation of the governments in the decision-making process of WADA. This was achieved through the Copenhagen Declaration on Anti-Doping in Sports.[113] The declaration was adopted in 2003 and signaled the support of the national governments to WADA.[114] It reiterated nation-state support for the WADA Code. It was essentially a political document, which stressed the need to have a harmonized anti-doping regime. The political commitments of the national governments, however, needed legal backing. That legal backing came in the form of the International Convention Against Doping in Sport.[115]

---

108 Lorenzo Casini, "Global Hybrid Public-private Bodies: The World Anti-Doping Agency (WADA)" (Global Administrative Law Conference, Geneva, 20–21 March 2009) www.iilj.org/wp-content/uploads/2017/03/Casini-Global-hybrid-public-private-bodies-2009.pdf (accessed 27 November 2018)

109 Ibid 8

110 Ibid 9

111 "World Anti-Doping Agency Chooses Canada for Headquarters" *CBC Television* (Montreal, 21 August 2001) www.cbc.ca/archives/entry/world-anti-doping-agency-chooses-canada-for-head quarters (accessed 27 November 2018)

112 David Howman, "Ten Years of WADA: Achievements, Challenges and The Way Forward" *Coventry* (2009) www.playthegame.org/uploads/media/David_Howman_-_Ten_years_of_WADA. pdf (accessed 27 November 2018)

113 "Copenhagen Declaration on Anti-Doping in Sport" www.wada-ama.org/sites/default/files/resources/files/WADA_Copenhagen_Declaration_EN.pdf (accessed 28 November 2018)

114 "Government Representation" www.wada-ama.org/en/government-representation (accessed 28 November 2018)

115 "International Convention Against Doping in Sport" (2005) www.wada-ama.org/sites/default/files/resources/files/UNESCO_Convention.pdf (accessed 28 November 2018)

The Copenhagen Declaration laid the framework for funding WADA. It was agreed that 50 percent of the funding would be from the governments. The percentage of the contribution was fixed by continent,[116] and the governments within the respective continents decided their individual share amongst themselves.[117] Accordingly, once the payment reached WADA, it invoiced each country individually.[118] The continental distribution, as was adopted in the Copenhagen Declaration and followed since, is: Africa, 0.5 percent; the Americas, 29 percent; Asia, 20.46 percent; Europe, 47.5 percent; Oceania, 2.54 percent.[119] It was agreed that the governments would align their domestic anti-doping policies with the WADA Code. Further, a continental distribution of WADA membership was agreed upon in the following order: four government nominees from the Americas, three from Africa, five from Europe, four from Asia and two from Oceania.[120] There was, in principal, agreement to provide legal, administrative and financial support to domestic doping control programmes.[121] The countries also agreed to cooperate in the testing and result management as part of doping control measures.[122] Finally, there was, in principal, agreement amongst the governments to continuously monitor compliances with the doping control commitments as undertaken.[123]

The International Convention Against Doping in Sport was adopted on 19 October 2005.[124] It was done under the aegis of the United Nations Educational, Scientific and Cultural Organization (UNESCO). Thus, formally, an intergovernmental organization became involved in anti-doping regulations for the first time. The Convention reflects the official stance of the nation-states on doping control. It embodies the legal commitments that the countries are voluntarily agreeing to doping control. It formalizes the process of international cooperation amongst nations against doping in sport. It also legitimizes the ethical principal of Olympism. Consequently, the moral argument against doping in the form of spirit of sport is officially recognized. Spirit of sport was transformed from informal rhetoric to an official stance of the international community. Finally, the Convention put the official seal on WADA and the WADA Code. Accordingly, the governments, through the ratification process, are liable for the implementation of the WADA Code in both letter and spirit.[125] The adoption and subsequent ratification of the Convention completed the process of legalizing the anti-doping regime.

---

116 "Copenhagen Declaration on Anti-Doping in Sport" (n 113) p. 4
117 "Funding by Governments" www.wada-ama.org/en/funding-by-governments (accessed 29 November 2018)
118 Ibid
119 "Copenhagen Declaration on Anti-Doping in Sport" (n 113) p. 4
120 Ibid 3
121 Ibid 5
122 Ibid
123 Ibid
124 "International Convention Against Doping in Sport" (n 115)
125 Ibid, Article 4

The Convention focuses on substance abuse only in the context of sport. Since the reference point continues to be the WADA Code, there is no reflection on the larger problem of drug addiction. Accordingly, the narrative that has been propagated by the IOC continues to hold sway. The Convention thus ensures that at the domestic level there will be conflicting policies on drug bans. The states commit themselves to treat the use of PEDs in sport as a problem separate from the use of narcotics in general. For example, alcohol consumption, which is otherwise permitted for the general public, was included in the 2004 Prohibited List.[126] Similarly, levmetamfetamine is used in certain inhalers for medicinal purposes, but it is on WADA's Prohibited List.[127] The Convention thus problematizes the anti-doping narrative. It completely ignores the existing contradiction in the anti-doping narrative which is premised on both health as well as moral grounds. The Convention does not require states to re-examine the question of prohibiting drugs in sport which are not inherently detrimental to health. The Convention furthers this contradiction by categorizing drug use in sport as illegitimate against the legitimate use of drugs for medicinal purpose.[128] The Convention thus creates no space for questioning the existing understanding of the anti-doping rationale. WADA and the WADA Code received official recognition at the international level through the Convention.

The Convention further ensures that the states commit themselves to tackle trafficking in PEDs.[129] Clearly, this is another instance of acknowledgement of the limitation that the IOC and its members have in doping control. The question then is why the governments and the IOC have not re-considered the parameters for doping control. The Convention did not add any novelty to the then-existing anti-doping philosophy. In the absence of self-introspection, the Convention, along with the Copenhagen Declaration became documents that legitimized WADA. Since then, WADA has grown in stature, secure in the knowledge of this legitimization. The approval of the international community in the form of governmental backing gave WADA the seal of authority. The Convention interestingly does not talk about any modicum of ensuring WADA's accountability. The responsibility of educating and training athletes and other sports administrators is left to the discretion of the state.[130] Further there is no scope of technology transfer or provision of assistance in developing adequate anti-doping frameworks in developing countries. Each state is left to its own with respect to developing a domestic anti-doping framework, from implementation to legislation. In short, the concerns of Third World countries are completely missing from this

---

126 The World Anti-Doping Code, "The 2004 Prohibited List" www.wada-ama.org/sites/default/files/resources/files/WADA_Prohibited_List_2004_EN.pdf (accessed 2 December 2018)
127 The World Anti-Doping Code, "International Standard-Prohibited List 2018" www.wada-ama.org/sites/default/files/prohibited_list_2018_en.pdf visited 2 December 2018
128 "International Convention Against Doping in Sport" (n 115) Article 7
129 Ibid
130 Ibid, Article 19

document. WADA was envisaged to be an autonomous body, outside the IOC, but not necessarily outside the influence of developed countries. The Convention came into force on 1 February 2007.[131]

The current representation within the WADA governing structure is: Africa, three members; the Americas, five members; Asia, four members; Europe, six members, and Oceania, two members.[132] This breakup indicates that the First World/developed countries continue to have an overbearing influence on WADA. Considering that WADA is a classic public–private partnership model, it impacts lives and livelihood beyond the mere private sphere. WADA is an example of international delegation of state authority to a specialized body.[133] The delegation is justified on the basis of expertise. Given that doping in sports is related to the larger issue of governance in sports, states prefer to not take on the responsibility directly. Further, because the anti-doping narrative affects only the athletes, it does not impinge on issues of sovereignty, as would be the case if citizens' rights were affected.[134] Armed with these advantages, WADA has ruled as a behemoth, enforcing its homogenized system without challenge. The concerns pertaining to WADA have therefore primarily been the concerns of a marginalized community, and more so when a subset of that community is from the developing countries.

Conclusion

From the beginning of its journey, WADA, and its predecessor the IOC Medical Commission, have authored an anti-doping narrative that ignores the realities of professionalism. Further, the justification of prohibiting PEDs is more ethical than practical. The current anti-doping narrative ignores the past, imagines the present as ideal and does not acknowledge the challenges of the future. The experiences of the discourse leading to the establishment of WADA reveals a process of self-denial. As will be seen in the next chapter, the government intrusions have not improved the scenario. On the contrary, WADA governance appears more as a saga of power play than a genuine concern for athletes. In this quagmire, the athletes are those who suffer the most. The next chapter reveals the murky scenario by analyzing the Russian doping scandal. This has been the biggest challenge that WADA has faced to date, and has led to existential questions for WADA.

Bibliography

Abbott, Karen, "The 1904 Olympic Marathon May Have Been the Strangest Ever' (2012) Smithsonian.com www.smithsonianmag.com/history/the-1904-olympic-marathon-may-have-been-the-strangest-ever-14910747/ (accessed 1 February 2018)

---

131 "Government Representation" (n 114)
132 Ibid
133 Abbas Ravjani, "The Court of Arbitration for Sport: A Subtle Form of International Delegation" (2008–2009) 2 *Journal of International Media and Entertainment Law* 241
134 Ibid

Barney, Robert K. "An Olympian Dilemma: Protection of Olympic Symbols" (2002) 10 (3) *Journal of Olympic History* 7–9 http://library.la84.org/SportsLibrary/JOH/JOHv10n3/JOHv10n3f.pdf (accessed 2 July 2018)

Beamish, Rob, "Chapter VII. Olympic Ideals Versus the Performance Imperative: The History of Canada's Anti-Doping Policies" in Lucie Thibault and Jean Harvey (ed.), *Sport Policy in Canada* (University of Ottawa Press, 2013) https://books.openedition.org/uop/711?lang=en (accessed 8 November 2018)

Beamish, Rob, *Steroids: A New Look at Performance Enhancing Drugs* (Praeger, 2011)

Beamish, Rob and Ian Ritchie, *Fastest, Highest, Strongest-a Critique of High-performance Sports* (Routledge, 2006)

Bertling, Christoph, "The Loss of Profit? The Rise of Professionalism in the Olympic Movement and the Consequences for National Sport Systems" (2007) 2 *Journal of Olympic History* 50 http://library.la84.org/SportsLibrary/JOH/JOHv15n2/JOHv15n2m.pdf (accessed 23 June 2018)

Boyd, Susan, "Pleasure and Pain-Representations of Illegal Drug Consumption, Addiction and Trafficking in Music, Film and Video" in Suzanne Fraser and David Moore (eds.), *The Drug Effect-Health, Crime and Society* (Cambridge University Press, 2011)

Brennan, Christine, "IOC Strips Johnson of Gold Medal in 100" *The Washington Post* (Washington, 27 September 1988) www.washingtonpost.com/archive/politics/1988/09/27/ioc-strips-johnson-of-gold-medal-in-100/9cd59877-87c4-44ec-9e96-69eb58f37fa2/?utm_term=.6c35b78036b1 (accessed 18 November 2018)

Brichford, Maynard, "Avery Brundage on Amateurism: Preaching and Practice" http://library.la84.org/SportsLibrary/ISOR/isor2010k.pdf (accessed 29 October 2018)

Brundage, Avery, "The IOC and Medical Problems" https://digital.la84.org/digital/collection/p17103coll1/id/28589/rec/1 (accessed 8 November 2018)

Calloway, Cab, "The Reefer Man (Original)" www.youtube.com/watch?v=svoSSdsNhtA

Casini, Lorenzo, "Global Hybrid Public-Private Bodies: The World Anti-Doping Agency (WADA)" (Global Administrative Law Conference, Geneva, 20–21 March 2009) www.iilj.org/wp-content/uploads/2017/03/Casini-Global-hybrid-public-private-bodies-2009.pdf (accessed 27 November 2018)

Chatziefstathiou, Dikaia, "The Changing Nature of the Ideology of Olympism in the Modern Olympic Era" https://dspace.lboro.ac.uk/dspace-jspui/bitstream/2134/2820/1/THESIS_FINAL%20090605_sb.pdf (accessed 23 June 2018)

Christensen, Peter, "The Drama about the Olympics in Rome" *Politiken* (2008) https://politiken.dk/kultur/boger/faglitteratur_boger/art4779455/Dramaet-om-OL-i-Rom (accessed 7 July 2018)

"Copenhagen Declaration on Anti-Doping in Sport" www.wada-ama.org/sites/default/files/resources/files/WADA_Copenhagen_Declaration_EN.pdf (accessed 28 November 2018)

Dimeo, Paul, *A History of Drug Use in Sports-1876–1976-Beyond Good and Evil* (Routledge, 2007)

Dimeo, Paul, "The Myth of Clean Sport and its Unintended Consequences" (2016) 4 (3–4) *Performance Enhancement and Health* 103 https://dspace.stir.ac.uk/bitstream/1893/23155/1/The%20Myth%20of%20Clean%20Sport%20%28with%20corrections%29%20updated.pdf (accessed 1 November 2018)

Dimeo, Paul, "The Truth About Knud: Revisiting an Anti-Doping Myth" *Sports Integrity Initiative* sportsintegrityintiative.com (accessed 25 October 2018)

Dimeo, Paul and Thomas Hunt, "Leading Anti-Doping in the IOC-the Ambiguous Role of Prince Alexandre de Merode" (2009) 17 (1) *Journal of Olympic History* 20 http://library.la84.org/SportsLibrary/JOH/JOHv17n1/JOHv17n1g.pdf (accessed 13 November 2018)

Dubin, Charles L. *Commission of Inquiry into the Use of Drugs and Banned Practices Intended to Increase Athletic Performance* (Canadian Government Publishing Centre, 1990) www.doping.nl/media/kb/3636/Dubin-report-1990-eng%20(S).pdf (accessed 16 November 2018)

"Extracts of the Minutes of the 65th Session of the International Olympic Committee Tehran, 6, 7, and 8 May 1967" http://library.la84.org/OlympicInformationCenter/OlympicReview/1967/BDCE98/BDCE98w.pdf (accessed 10 November 2018)

Fitzgerald, Ella, "Wacky Dust" www.youtube.com/watch?v=RjRcKq38-IY (accessed 7 February 2018)

"Funding by Governments" www.wada-ama.org/en/funding-by-governments (accessed 29 November 2018)

Gleaves, John, "Doped Professionals and Clean Amateurs: Amateurism's Influence on the Modern Philosophy of Anti-Doping" (2011) 38 (2) *Journal of Sport History* 248

Gordon, Aaron, "The Morality Myth Behind the Modern Anti-Doping Movement" (2017) *Vice Sports* sports.vice.com (accessed 27 October 2018)

"Government Representation" www.wada-ama.org/en/government-representation (accessed 28 November 2018)

Greenhow, Annette, "Drug Use in Sport: What's Changed?" (2010), 16 (2) *The National Legal Eagle* http://epublications.bond.edu.au/cgi/viewcontent.cgi?article=1152&context=nle (accessed 1 February 2018)

Hacke, Detlef, "From Festina to Team Telekom/Team T-Mobile – Doping Scandals in Cycling" www.uni-freiburg.de/universitaet/einzelgutachten/symposium-freiburg-2011-hacke.pdf (accessed 21 November 2018)

Hand Book of the International Amateur Athletic Federation, 1927–28, Section 13 and Section 22 www.iaaf.org/news/news/a-piece-of-anti-doping-history-iaaf-handbook (accessed 1 February 2018)

Handbook of the International Amateur Athletic Federation, 1927–28 www.iaaf.org/download/download?filename=bd61cf34-14b2-4dfc-9745-de91; www.iaaf.org/news/news/a-piece-of-anti-doping-history-iaaf-handbook (accessed 24 October 2018)

Hanstad, Dag Vidar, Andy Smith and Ivan Waddington, "The Establishment of the World Anti-Doping Agency: A Study of the Management of Organizational Change and Unplanned Outcomes" www.researchgate.net/profile/Ivan_Waddington/publication/233540368_The_Establishment_of_the_World_Anti-Doping_Agency_A_Study_of_the_Management_of_Organizational_Change_and_Unplanned_Outcomes/links/55ad1b7008aee079921d510e/The-Establishment-of-the-World-Anti-Doping-Agency-A-Study-of-the-Management-of-Organizational-Change-and-Unplanned-Outcomes.pdf (accessed 23 November 2018)

Henne, Kathryn E. "The Origins of the International Olympic Committee Medical Commission and Its Technocratic Regime: An Historiographic Investigation of Anti-Doping Regulation and Enforcement in International Sport" www.academia.edu/530687/The_Origins_of_the_International_Olympic_Committee_Medical_Commission_and_its_Technocratic_Regime_An_Historiographic_Investigation_of_Anti-Doping_ (accessed 15 November 2018)

Hersh, Philip, "IOC Anti-Doping 'Declaration' Is No Victory for Samaranch" *Chicago Tribune* (Chicago, 5 February 1999) www.chicagotribune.com/news/ct-xpm-1999-02-05-9902050084-story.html (accessed 23 November 2018)

Hobberman, John, "Backtalk: Offering the Illusion of Reform on Drugs" *The New York Times* (New York, 10 January 1999)

Hobberman, John, *Mortal Engines-the Science of Performance and the Dehumanization of Sport* (The Blackburn Press, 1992)

Hobberman, John, *Testosterone Dreams: Rejuvenation, Aphrodisia, Doping* (University of California Press, 2005)

Howman, David, "Ten Years of WADA: Achievements, Challenges and the Way Forward" *Coventry* (2009) www.playthegame.org/uploads/media/David_Howman_-_Ten_years_of_WADA.pdf (accessed 27 November 2018)

"International Convention Against Doping in Sport" (2005) www.wada-ama.org/sites/default/files/resources/files/UNESCO_Convention.pdf (accessed 28 November 2018)

International Olympic Committee, "Medical Commission-Overview of the Content of the Archives Concerning the History, Missions and Activities of the IOC Medical Commission from 1936 to 1995" https://stillmed.olympic.org/media/Document%20Library/OlympicOrg/Olympic-Studies-Centre/List-of-Resources/Resources-available/Archives/EN-Medical-Commission.pdf (accessed 8 November 2018)

Johnson, Mark, *Spitting in The Soup-inside the Dirty Game of Doping in Sports* (VeloPress, 2016)

Joy, Bernard, *Forward, Arsenal! The First Detailed History of Arsenal Football Club 1886–1953* (GCR Books, 2009)

Kremenik, Michael, Sho Onodera, Mitsushiro Nagao, Osamu Yuzuki and Shozo Yonetani, "A Historical Timeline of Doping in the Olympics (Part 1 1896–1968)" (2006) 12 (1) *Kawasaki Journal of Medical Welfare* 1919 www.kawasaki-m.ac.jp/soc/mw/journal/en/2006-e12-1/01_kremenik.pdf (accessed 8 November 2018)

"Lausanne Declaration on Doping in Sport-adopted by the World Conference on Doping in Sport 4 February 1999, Lausanne, Switzerland" www.wada-ama.org/sites/default/files/resources/files/lausanne_declaration_on_doping_in_sport.pdf (accessed 24 November 2018)

Ljungqvist, Arne, "Brief History of Anti-Doping" in O. Rabin and Y. Pitsiladis (eds.), *Acute Topics in Anti-Doping. Medicine and Sport Science* 62 (Basel, Karger, 2017) www.karger.com/WebMaterial/ShowFileCache/877472 (accessed 9 November 2018)

Llewellyn, Matthew P. and John T. Gleaves, "The Rise of the 'Shamateur' The International Olympic Committee and the Preservation of the Amateur Idea" http://library.la84.org/SportsLibrary/ISOR/isor2012h.pdf (accessed 3 July 2018)

Llewellyn, Matthew P. and John T. Gleaves, "The Rise of the Shamateur The International Olympic Committee, Broken-Time Payments, and the Preservation of the Amateur Ideal, 1925–1930" (2014) XXIII *Olympika* 1 http://library.la84.org/SportsLibrary/Olympika/Olympika_2014/olympika2014c.pdf (25 June 2018)

Longman, Jere, "Olympics: I.O.C. Drug Chief Calls for Shift in Bans" *The New York Times* (New York, 29 January 1999)

Lucas, Charles J. P. *The Olympic Games-1904* (St. Louis, MO, Woodward & Tiernan Printing Co., 1905) http://library.la84.org/6oic/OfficialReports/1904/1904lucas.pdf (accessed 2 February 2018)

Mackay, Duncan, "Samaranch to Lead Drug Agency" *The Guardian* (London, 2 February 1999) www.theguardian.com/sport/1999/feb/02/samaranch-head-anti-doping-agency (accessed 22 November 2018)

Maloney, Patrick, "Ben Johnson Scandal/ 25 Years Later" *Ottawa Sun* (Ottawa, 22 September 2013) https://ottawasun.com/2013/09/22/ben-johnson-scandal-25-years-later/wcm/7a445688-6861-40b3-a21f-665404f11699 (accessed 16 November 2018)

Mann, Andrea, "September 27, 1988: Ben Johnson Is Stripped of His Olympic Gold Medal After Failing Drugs Test the Most Famous Men's 100m Final in the History of the Olympics Became the Most Infamous When Canadian Sprinter Ben Johnson Was Found Guilty of Taking Steroids" *BT* (Montreal, 26 September 2018) http://home. bt.com/news/on-this-day/september-27-1988-ben-johnson-is-stripped-of-his-olympic-gold-medal-after-failing-drugs-test-11364007354384 (accessed 16 November 2018)

Mignon, Patrick, "The Tour de France and the Doping Issue" (2003) 20 (2) *International Journal of the History of Sport*, Taylor Francis (Routledge) 227 https://hal-insep.archives-ouvertes.fr/hal-01697488/document (accessed 8 November 2018)

Møller, Verner, "Knud Enemark Jensen's Death During the 1960 Rome Olympics: A Search for Truth?" (2005) 25 (3) *Sport in History* 452 www.academia.dk/Blog/wp-content/uploads/VernerMoller_KnudEnemark.pdf (accessed 7 July 2018)

Moore, Jack, "Throwback Thursday: Ben Johnson at the Seoul Olympics, and the Doping Race That Never Ends Ben Johnson's 100m Dash Victory and Subsequent Steroid Bust at the 1988 Summer Games Was a Watershed Moment for Anti-Doping Activists, But to What End?" *Vice Sports* (Montreal, 24 September 2015) https://sports.vice.com/en_ca/article/53v7xd/throwback-thursday-ben-johnson-at-the-seoul-olympics-and-the-doping-race-that-never-ends (accessed 16 November 2018)

Murray, James, "Olympians Put Avery Brundage on the Spot" *Sports Illustrated Vault* (1956) www.si.com/vault/1956/08/27/584401/olympians-put-avery-brundage-on-the-spot (accessed 30 October 2018)

Obituary, "Marc Hodler: Exposed Scandal in Selection of Olympics' Host Cities" *Associated Press* (Lausanne, 20 October 2006) www.washingtonpost.com/wp-dyn/content/article/2006/10/19/AR2006101901725.html (accessed 22 November 2018)

Obituary, "Prince Alexandre de Mrode" *The Telegraph* (London, 27 November 2002) www.telegraph.co.uk/news/obituaries/1414375/Prince-Alexandre-de-Merode.html (accessed 13 November 2018)

Official Bulletin of the International Olympic Committee, "Minutes of the Meeting of the Executive Committee Paris 8th August 1927" http://library.la84.org/OlympicInformationCenter/OlympicReview/1927/BODE8/BODE8g.pdf (accessed 3 July 2018)

Olympic Charter, "Fundamental Principles of Olympism" https://stillmed.olympic.org/media/Document%20Library/OlympicOrg/General/EN-Olympic-Charter.pdf#_ga=2.146302775.2066783038.1497077375-1924997101.1497077375 (accessed 29 May 2017)

Olympic Charter, 1938, Rule 17 https://stillmed.olympic.org/media/Document%20Library/OlympicOrg/Olympic-Studies-Centre/List-of-Resources/Official-Publications/Olympic-Charters/EN-1938-Olympic-Charter-Olympic-Rules.pdf#_ga=2.140216692.692104528.1529993269-130387347.1524895071 (accessed 25 June 2018)

Prokop, Ludwig, "Drug Abuse in International Athletics" (1975) 3 (2) *Journal of Sports Medicine* 85

Prokop, Ludwig, "Doping" www.cycling4fans.de/index.php?id=5302 (accessed 2 November 2018)

Ravjani, Abbas, "The Court of Arbitration for Sport: A Subtle Form of International Delegation" (2008–2009) 2 *Journal of International Media and Entertainment Law*

Report and Restatement of the Question of Doping, presented at the Moscow International Olympic Committee Session in June 1962 by Dr J. Ferreira Santos titled "Doping" http://library.la84.org/OlympicInformationCenter/OlympicReview/1963/BDCE81/BDCE81u.pdf (accessed 2 November 2018)

Ritchie, Ian, "Before and After 1968: Reconsidering the Introduction of Drug Testing in the Olympic Games" in Stephen Wagg (ed.), *Myths and Milestones in the History of Sport* (Palgrave Macmillan, 2011)

Ritchie, Ian, "Cops and Robbers? The Roots of Anti-Doping Policies in Olympic Sport" (2016) 9 (6) (Origins) *Current Events in Historical Perspective*

Ritchie, Ian, "Understanding Performance Enhancing Substances and Sanctions Against their Use from the Perspective of History" in Verner Moller, Ivan Waddington and John M. Hobberman (eds.), *Routledge Handbook of Drugs and Sport* (Routledge, 2015)

Teetzel, Sarah, "'The Road to WADA', Cultural Relations Old and New: The Transitory Olympic Ethos" (2004) *Seventh International Symposium for Olympic Research* 213 https://digital.la84.org/digital/collection/p17103coll10/id/13553/rec/4 (accessed 22 November 2018)

Waddington, I., D. Malcolm, M. Roderick and R. Naik, "Drug Use in English Professional Football" (2005) 39 (18) *British Journal of Sports Medicine* www.bjsportmed.com/cgi/content/full/39/4/e18; doi: 10.1136/bjsm.2004.012468 (accessed 7 February 2018)

Weed Smoker's Dream, "Harlem Hamfats'" www.youtube.com/watch?v=uyjW8FTGxbI

Wilson, Wayne and Edward Derse (eds.), *Doping in Elite Sport-the Politics of Drugs in the Olympic Movement* (Human Kinetics Publishers, 2001)

"World: Europe French Doping Crackdown" *BBC* (London, 19 November 1998) http://news.bbc.co.uk/2/hi/europe/217845.stm (accessed 23 November 2018)

"World Anti-Doping Agency Chooses Canada for Headquarters" *CBC Television* (Montreal, 21 August 2001) www.cbc.ca/archives/entry/world-anti-doping-agency-chooses-canada-for-headquarters (accessed 27 November 2018)

World Anti-Doping Code, "International Standard-Prohibited List 2018" www.wada-ama.org/sites/default/files/prohibited_list_2018_en.pdf visited 2 December 2018

World Anti-Doping Code, "The 2004 Prohibited List" www.wada-ama.org/sites/default/files/resources/files/WADA_Prohibited_List_2004_EN.pdf (accessed 2 December 2018)

Yesalis, Charles E. and Michael S. Bahrke, "History of Doping in Sport" (2002) 24 (1) *International Sports Studies* http://library.la84.org/SportsLibrary/ISS/ISS2401/ISS2401e.pdf (accessed 8 February 2018)

Yttergren, Leif, "J. Sigfrid Edstrom and the Nurmi Affair of 1932: The Struggle of the Amateur Fundamentalists Against Professionalism in the Olympic Movement" (2007) 15 (3) *Journal of Olympic History* 21 library.la84.org/SportsLibrary/JOH/JOHv15n3/JOHv15n3h.pdf (accessed 24 October 2018)

Chapter 2

The Russian doping scandal and the WADA Code

A flawed deal for a developing country/non-elite athlete?

Introduction

The emphasis on self-affirmation of the current anti-doping regime, as mapped out in the previous chapter, has not prevented sporting scandals from testing the viability of this strategy. While the Tour de France scandal laid the foundation of the 2003 WADA Code, the Russian doping scandal has raised doubts about the effectiveness of the 2015 WADA Code. The reports on the manner by which Russia conned the entire system and won medals has brought forth the limitations of WADA. Lack of monitoring and enforcement mechanisms appear to be WADA's biggest problems. The reports prepared by WADA's Independent Commission as well as the Independent Person report are filled with the manner by which Russia manipulated each and every existing WADA-enforced system. State-sanctioned doping may be used as an argument to explain the Russian scandal, but the larger question is what WADA could have done to prevent it. Furthermore, the 2015 Code incorporates certain features that make the application of No Fault or No Significant Fault more flexible. The point then is to understand whether the changes brought to bear are good enough to prevent future scandals. It is also important to consider WADA's ability to prevent or detect doping at a mass scale by a country as powerful as Russia. The other concern is the state of denial in acknowledging that there needs to be a revisiting of the existing philosophy that is used to design all anti-doping programmes. The Russian scandal also raises concerns that poor and non-elite athletes are vulnerable under a system that can easily be manipulated by the elite and powerful. The Russian scandal creates an urgency to revamp the WADA system, for it has proven to be too elitist in terms of accessibility to justice.

Winners take it all! The Germans unmask the Russians

It was the 2014 Sochi Winter Olympic Games, and Russia was enjoying the glory, not only as a host, but also as the winner of the highest number of gold medals.

Russia thus topped the medal tally, ahead of the US.[1] Soon though the glory turned into a nightmare for all concerned when in December 2014 the German public broadcaster ARD aired a documentary on Russian doping.[2] The documentary was filmed by Hajo Seppelt, who became interested in the matter after receiving several e-mails.[3] In particular Seppelt became curious about an e-mail sent by Vitaly Stepanov and his wife Yuliya. Vitaliy was working with the Russian Anti-Doping Agency (RUSADA). Yuliya was an 800 m sprinter who, at the time of the filming of the documentary, was under suspension for doping. They revealed to Seppelt the elaborate but secret Russian doping programme. The coaches trained the athletes to take drugs, hammering into them that PEDs were the only option for winning. PEDs like erythropoietin (EPO) were easily available without a prescription. Doping control officers were bribed into ignoring the use of PEDs by Russian athletes. Russian athletes were asked to keep clean samples to switch with contaminated ones to avoid detection. Seppelt's interview revealed that 99 percent of Russian athletes were using PEDs. The system was managed by the Russian coaches and highly placed sports officials.

The athletes were left with no option but to agree since the entire Russian sports hierarchy, including the Russian Ministry of Sport and the Russian Athletic Federation, was involved. Individual athletes were given detailed schedules covering what kinds of banned drugs they were to be given along with the dosage and timing. The objective was to avoid detection at international competitions, and, in case someone was caught, to drop that athlete from the list and start fresh with a new person. Further, the Ministry of Sport and anti-doping officials monitored the tests performed by RUSADA. In all cases where the sample of a medal hopeful or a potential winner or an established star athlete tested positive, the test was covered up. Only a few athletes who were on the fringes of success and fame were reported, thus putting up a show of transparency. The involvement of the Russian government extended to the point of opening and checking the samples before they were transported outside the country. WADA did not protest, nor was there any widespread action on the part of IOC or IAAF or other International Federations. Russia legalized this intervention through legislative enactment. Contrary to the commitments made under the International Convention, Russia was interfering with doping control and manipulating it.

1 R. Cory Smith, "Olympic Medal Count 2014: Final Standings and Sochi Medal Tally for Each Country" *Bleacher Report* (2014) https://bleacherreport.com/articles/1970880-olympic-medal-count-2014-final-standings-and-sochi-medal-tally-for-each-country (accessed 2 December 2018)

2 Prospero, "'Icarus' Reveals the Mastermind Behind Russia's Doping Programme" *The Economist* (London, 8 August 2017) www.economist.com/prospero/2017/08/08/icarus-reveals-the-master mind-behind-russias-doping-programme (accessed 2 December 2018)

3 Lucky Loser Tennis, "The Secrets of Doping: How Russia Makes Its Winners – H. Seppelt (ARD – 2014)" *YouTube* (2015) www.youtube.com/watch?v=iu9B-ty9JCY&t=7s (accessed 2 December 2018)

Russian national coaches ensured that there was a proper screening process of the athletes before any international competition. The purpose of the screening process was to ensure that none of the athletes tested positive in the concerned international competition. Anyone who did test positive never accompanied the team, even if selected for the competition. That way Russia ensured that there was no detection in the international competition. Seppelt got transcripts of telephone conversations of star Russian athlete Maria Savinova. She was the European and World Champion of the 800 m. She did not test positive for PEDs. In her conversation, as recorded and revealed by the transcript, she admits to regularly using PEDs. She had no qualms and accepted that the only way to win was through drugs. She acknowledged the role of her coaches and the Russian system that helped her avoid detection. Her conversation reveals the important role played by a WADA-accredited laboratory in avoiding detection. Interestingly Seppelt's investigation reveals that WADA had been aware of irregularities taking place in the Russian laboratory. However, they failed to initiate any steps to inquire into the same.

The most WADA did was threaten to revoke the lab's accreditation, which, under the existing rules, is the maximum punishment. WADA's threat however did not materialize, and the lab continued to enjoy accreditation. Seppelt met the director of the Russian lab, Grigoriy Rodchenkov. As will be seen later, he was one of the biggest players in implementing the Russian doping programme. However, he bluntly denied any knowledge or existence of any organized doping programme to Seppelt. Seppelt's investigation also points fingers at the IAAF and the involvement of its officials in the Russian cover-up. Seppelt found that the president of the Russian Athletic Federation had taken bribes from athletes to cover up the use of PEDs. Interestingly, even though the IAAF had grounds to suspect manipulation, it did not take any action, nor did it initiate an inquiry. Not surprisingly, Valentin Balakhnichev, the president of the Russian Athletic Federation, kept denying his involvement in the doping cover-up when asked about it by Seppelt. Balakhnichev was also the treasurer of the IAAF, thus holding a post of importance within the International Federation. Clearly, the entire Russian doping programme was facilitated by the presence of people guided by self-interest.

WADA did receive a large number of e-mails containing information about the Russian doping scandal.[4] However it did not act upon them. On the revelations being made by Hajo Seppelt, WADA went on the defensive by citing its inherent lack of authority to initiate suo moto investigations. However, that cannot be an excuse not to exercise the powers that it had viz. to cancel the accreditation of the Russian laboratory. Further it could have ensured proper result management, including sample handling and testing. That an IAAF official was

4 Eddie Pells, "60 Minutes: WADA Received 200 Emails from Whistleblower About Russian Doping Scandal" *The Associated Press* (New York, 9 May 2016) www.cbc.ca/sports/olympics/russia-doping-scandal-whistleblower-1.3572938 (accessed 2 December 2018)

involved should have led WADA to insist on coordinated action in the matter. Unfortunately, WADA, as noted in the previous chapter, is not outside the influence of sporting powerhouses like Russia, hence taking any initiative against such a powerful nation was clearly not desirable. Seppelt's investigations ignited public sentiment against the organized doping programme. The public image of WADA, the IOC and the other international sports organizations took a beating. Pressure mounted on WADA to take action. Accordingly, WADA invoked its power under Article 5.8 of the 2015 Code[5] and tasked Dick Pound with leading an Independent Commission. The German journalist not only unmasked the Russians, he also led WADA to conduct an investigation at an unprecedented scale.[6]

The Independent Commission report and WADA – decoding the elitist paradigm

The Independent Commission (hereinafter called the IC) was slated to begin its work on 11 December 2014, the date of its appointment. The IC was composed of three members: Richard W. Pound, QC (chair), Richard H. McLaren and Günter Younger. Its mandate was to investigate the allegations raised in the ARD documentary. The suspects were both the Russian Sports Federations as well as the IAAF. The terms of reference further authorized the IC to investigate allegations of infractions against other International Federations and anti-doping organizations. The IC was required to submit its report to WADA by 31 December 2015.[7] Subsequent ARD documentaries about large-scale doping within athletics[8] extended the mandate of the IC. Accordingly, on 17 August 2015 WADA issued an addendum to investigate specifically the role of the IAAF in major cover-ups of doping in athletics.[9] The reference point of the IC, as per this addendum,

5 WADA Code 2015 Article 5.8, [5.8 Investigations and Intelligence Gathering Anti-Doping Organizations shall ensure they are able to do each of the following, as applicable and in accordance with the International Standard for Testing and Investigations:5.8.1 Obtain, assess and process anti-doping intelligence from all available sources to inform the development of an effective, intelligent and proportionate test distribution plan, to plan Target Testing, and/or to form the basis of an investigation into a possible anti-doping rule violation(s)] www.wada-ama.org/sites/default/files/resources/files/wada-2015-world-anti-doping-code.pdf (accessed 3 December 2018). The 2015 Code came into effect on 1 January 2015

6 WADA, "WADA Announces Details of Independent Commission" (2014) www.wada-ama.org/en/media/news/2014-12/wada-announces-details-of-independent-commission (accessed 3 December 2018)

7 WADA, "Independent Commission-Terms of Reference" (2015) www.wada-ama.org/sites/default/files/wada independent-commission-terms-of-reference-2015-jan-en.pdf (accessed 3 December 2018)

8 Lucky Loser Tennis, "H. Seppelt – The Secrets of Doping – the Shadowy World of Athletics – ARD 2015 – English" You Tube (2015) www.youtube.com/watch?v=nIkiC3iT0GA (accessed 2 December 2018)

9 WADA, "Independent Commission Terms of Reference (Addendum)" (2015) www.wada-ama.org/sites/default/files/resources/files/wada-independent-commission-tor-addendum-en.pdf (accessed 3 December 2018)

was to obtain the database of blood values of elite athletes, which were leaked to Seppelt. As Seppelt reveals in the 2015 ARD documentary, the database was huge and indicated widespread doping in athletics. The data revealed that high-performing athletes from Kenya had suspicious blood values.[10]

Interestingly, the additional terms of reference limited the scope of the IC to review the role of WADA in the failure of the IAAF. The rationale given was that WADA was required to only regulate and monitor anti-doping programmes. In other words, the implementation of the anti-doping programme at the ground level was the responsibility of the IAAF and its domestic representative federations.[11] The IC completed its investigations and submitted its report on 9 November 2015.[12] As per the findings of the IC, winning at all costs was behind the Russian doping programme. What needs to be noted is that the mentality to win is not a recent phenomenon. It is acknowledged by the IC to be closely linked with the need to assert political power and prestige. Sport provides that avenue, and hence doping is tolerated and encouraged.[13] Thus, for the IC doping is as an example of deviance. The reference to this argument is taken form the WADA Code. The Code identifies spirit of sport as the rationale that legitimizes anti-doping measures.[14] According to this, spirit of sport is

> the celebration of the human spirit, body and mind, and is reflected in values we find in and through sport, including:
>
> - Ethics, fair play and honesty
> - Health
> - Excellence in performance
> - Character and education
> - Fun and joy
> - Teamwork
> - Dedication and commitment
> - Respect for rules and laws
> - Respect for self and other Participants
> - Courage
> - Community and solidarity
>
> Doping is fundamentally contrary to the spirit of sport.[15]

10 Lucky Loser Tennis (n 8)
11 WADA, "Statement Regarding Extended Mandate of Independent Commission" (2015) www.wada-ama.org/en/media/news/2015-08/statement-regarding-extended-mandate-of-independent-commission (accessed 3 December 2018)
12 WADA Independent Commission, "The Independent Commission Report #1 Final Report" *The Independent Investigation* (2015) www.wada-ama.org/sites/default/files/resources/files/wada_independent_commission_report_1_en.pdf (accessed 3 December 2018)
13 Ibid 76–77
14 WADA Code 2015, "Fundamental Rationale for The World Anti-Doping Code" www.wada-ama.org/sites/default/files/resources/files/wada-2015-world-anti-doping-code.pdf (accessed 3 December 2018)
15 Ibid

The IC effectively ignores the fact that the use of PEDs was historically acceded to by the IOC and its members (as discussed in Chapter 1). Having thus built the narrative of a zero-tolerance policy towards doping, the IC goes on to evaluate the role of different players in the Russian doping saga.

The IC identified and affirmed that the Russian lab at Moscow, accredited by WADA, miserably failed in its role. Lab director Grigory Rodchenko led the manipulation of doping results.[16] The IC found that the Russian government influenced the process of sample testing and result management. There was evidence of the destruction of samples and elaborate efforts to cover up doping by Russian athletes. The IC found that Rodchenko took bribes to ensure that the athletes were never detected. The IC found that during the Sochi Winter Olympics the independence of the Moscow laboratory was compromised.[17] Doping control during the Sochi Olympics was thus compromised, and the results were managed in favour of Russian athletes. The IC found existence of a second laboratory that was suspected to be used for destruction of samples. Advance notice of out-of-competition tests was provided, in clear violation of WADA Code.[18] RUSADA failed to enforce the Code provisions pertaining to whereabouts filing.[19] There were a large number of whereabouts filing failures that were not acted upon. There were many instances of missed tests and false identities being given to evade testing. Bribing the Doping Control Officers (DCOs) associated with RUSADA was routine and an institutionalized practice to avoid detection. There was evidence of intimidation of the DCOs and their family members by the Russian State to ensure effective cover up of doping.[20]

RUSADA permitted sanctioned athletes to compete during the period of sanctions in violation of the Code. RUSADA was found to have colluded with coaches in ensuring effective cover-up of anti-doping violations. RUSADA was found to have compromised its role as an impartial and independent anti-doping agency. RUSADA was thus actively promoting the elaborate cover-up scheme to enable Russian athletes to freely use PEDs.[21] The All Russian Athletics Federation (ARAF) was non-cooperative with the IC investigators throughout the inquiry.[22] Investigations by the IC revealed that the ARAF promoted a culture of doping complicit with coaches and other highly placed officials. This culture left the athletes with no choice but to accept the doping programme or face the prospect of losing out on the chance to compete. The ARAF was found to have deliberately ignored cases of abnormal blood values, allowing athletes with abnormal blood values to compete freely.[23] The IC investigations revealed that the ARAF's chief medical officer was openly violating the Code. In addition, the president of the

16 WADA Independent Commission (n 12) 12
17 Ibid 13–14
18 Ibid 15
19 Ibid 16
20 Ibid
21 Ibid 19
22 Ibid 19–20
23 Ibid 22

ARAF at the time, Balakhnichev, was also responsible for the Code violations that took place under his leadership. Coaches were found to have been involved in trafficking with the support of the ARAF. Balakhnichev also colluded with the director of the Moscow laboratory, Rodchenko, to swap dirty samples with clean samples. They took bribes from the athletes for the same.[24]

Russian sports officials were expected to protect athletes from any consequence of doping. ARAF Medical Commission Chief Dr Sergey Portugalov not only encouraged doping but also personally injected athletes with drugs. Dr Portugalov was actively involved in covering up doping violations of athletes in return for a percentage of their winnings.[25] The Russian Ministry of Sport was actively involved and encouraged the doping programme. The IC investigations revealed that the Ministry of Sport clearly influenced the way RUSADA and the Moscow laboratory functioned.[26] The IC investigations found that there were well-planned and organized violations of IAAF rules and WADA Code by the IAAF officials. The IAAF officials colluded with the ARAF officials to provide cover to Russian athletes. The IAAF was lax in following up with the ARAF for the latter's inaction.[27] Overall, the IAAF was contributory to the smooth running of the Russian doping programme. The IC thus found all the stakeholders guilty of allowing the Russian doping programme to be in place for a long time. It reveals a clear influence of power and money at play. It reveals that a politically powerful country can pull strings to con the system. It reveals that elite athletes and rich countries can conveniently ignore the strict WADA Code. The institutions that have continuously propagated and institutionalized the concept of spirit of sport are the ones to violate it. Unfortunately, the sporting world being a hegemony of the powerful is a classic example of conflict of interest.

The International Sports Federations are expected to take actions against their own. There is no scope of an entirely independent agency. As the Russian scandal reveals, WADA's structure as an independent agency is not truly independent. Powerful countries are there to control the decision-making processes of WADA. The IOC and its member federations constitute the other half controlling WADA. In such a scenario, the vested interests of the elite will determine when a scandal will be detected and acted upon. It's always a reactionary process, and there are no preemptive measures that appear to be taken. The limitations of WADA were highlighted by the IC in its report. As per IC, WADA faces an immense financial crunch in its mission of conducting anti-doping activities.[28] Considering that WADA is dependent on the IOC and the governments for its funding, it is their combined decision which will determine its efficiency. The IC recommended that it should be mandatory for all to feed data into the

24 Ibid 23
25 WADA Independent Commission (n 12) 25
26 Ibid 28
27 Ibid 29–30
28 Ibid 31

Anti-Doping Administration & Management System (ADAMS). This would enable WADA to have better control over the anti-doping monitoring process. The IC recommended that WADA needed to seriously undertake its role of conducting educational programmes on anti-doping regulations. In addition, WADA was also expected to ensure compliance by the signatories. The IC acknowledged that the members in charge of WADA governance were primarily led by their self-interest.[29]

Agendas driven by self-interest create hurdles in the way of WADA effectively implementing and taking strong measures against infractions. Further, the IC notes that the stakeholders are not proactive in strengthening the hands of WADA. On the contrary, the IC notes that the stakeholders have been recalcitrant in strictly implementing the WADA Code.[30] Further, WADA was also found to be lax in ensuring compliance from signatories. WADA, as per the IC report, was found to have the requisite expertise to implement the Code. It was also acknowledged that WADA was to have created an awareness about the need to protect clean athletes.[31] However WADA was found to have no control over the functioning of the accredited laboratories, the third-party contracts of these laboratories or the problems faced by the DCOs. Finally, the IC recommended the need to develop an effective whistle-blower assistance and protection programme, incentivizing the whistle-blowers to cooperate with WADA.[32] The IC's findings clearly indicate that the anti-doping narrative is driven more by politics then by any desire to take action. Hence, for the elites of world sports, there is nothing to fear. WADA will be tamed as and when required in the interest of the elite athlete.

The IC's findings also underline that, irrespective of the stringency of anti-doping measures, doping cannot be rooted out. Unfortunately, there is no larger discussion on the need to re-visit the spirit of sport philosophy. Hence, any possibility of re-orienting the discussion is clearly ruled out. The second part of the IC report was submitted on 14 January 2016.[33] The report implicates the then IAAF President Lamine Diack of corruption. He was found to have personal knowledge of the Russian doping scheme. Thus, the anti-doping programme was manipulated to suit the interests of Russia and IAAF officials.[34] The IAAF and ARAF were found to be closely connected with running the doping programme. Balakhnichev being both the president of the ARAF and the treasurer of IAAF at the same point in time complicated matters. Thus, the IAAF was equally

29 Ibid 32
30 Ibid
31 WADA Independent Commission (n 12)
32 Ibid 33
33 WADA Independent Commission, "The Independent Commission Report #2" *Independent Commission Investigation* (2016) www.wada-ama.org/sites/default/files/resources/files/wada_independent_commission_report_2_2016_en_rev.pdf (accessed 3 December 2018)
34 Ibid 11

responsible for the ARAF's faults and laxity.[35] The IAAF was found to be a willing partner of Russia and shielded its doping activities.[36] This is another example of the structural impediments that exist within sports governing bodies and WADA, making it impossible to make any independent decision on anti-doping measures. Article 20 of the Code elaborately points out the roles and responsibility of all the stakeholders viz. the IOC; the International Federations (IFs); the National Anti-Doping Organizations; the International Paralympic Committee; the National Olympic Committee and National Paralympic Committee; the Major Event Organizations and WADA, are to play. However, the experiences and findings of the IC reveal that these are practices that are difficult to enforce. The IC reports reveal the depth of influence and control that elite and developed countries have, thereby converting the WADA Code into a pro-elite document.

The IOC and the Russian scandal – turning a blind eye?

Following the publication of the IC reports, Grigory Rodchenko, the director of the Moscow lab implicated in the IC report and the ARD documentary as a key player, made startling revelations. In 2016, Rodchenko turned whistle-blower, having defected to the US in 2015.[37] In his interview given to the *New York Times* on 12 May 2016, Rodchenko claimed that the 2014 Sochi Olympics were manipulated by Russia, and that most of the medal winners from Russia were doped and that the Russian results in the 2014 Olympics were the outcome of an elaborate state-sponsored doping scheme.[38] Rodchenko summed up his take on the Russian doping scheme by stating that "People are celebrating Olympic champion winners, but we are sitting crazy and replacing their urine."[39] This interview led WADA to constitute an independent investigation into the allegations pertaining to the 2014 Sochi Winter Olympics.[40] On 18 May 2016 the Independent Person (IP), Prof Richard H. McLaren, was appointed to investigate the allegations. Prof McLaren submitted his report on 16 July 2016.[41] The report

---

35 Ibid 12–13

36 Ibid 41–48

37 Jada Yuan, "How Bryan Fogel Accidentally Documented the Russian Olympic Doping Scandal-and Helped Its Key Player Escape to the United States" *Vulture* (2017) www.vulture.com/2017/12/icarus-bryan-fogel-russia-doping-scandal-olympics-netflix.html (accessed 3 December 2018)

38 Rebecca R. Ruiz and Michael Schwirtz, "Russian Insider Says State-run Doping Fueled Olympic Gold" *The New York Times* (New York, 12 May 2016) www.nytimes.com/2016/05/13/sports/russia-doping-sochi-olympics-2014.html (accessed 3 December 2018)

39 Ibid

40 WADA, "Independent Investigation into the Sochi Allegations Made by Grigory Rodchenkov" (2016) www.wada-ama.org/sites/default/files/resources/files/wada-independent-investigation-of-g-rodchenkov-allegations-tor-en_0.pdf (accessed 4 December 2018)

41 Richard H. Mclaren Independent Person, "The Independent Person Report" *WADA Investigation of Sochi Allegations* (2016) www.wada-ama.org/sites/default/files/resources/files/20160718_ip_report_newfinal.pdf (accessed 3 December 2018)

found that the Sochi laboratory, accredited by WADA, was used to swap the dirty sample with a clean sample.[42] The Russian Federal Security Service (FSB) was involved in tampering with the bottles containing the sample and switching the same.[43] Initially under the direction of the Russian State, the Moscow laboratory developed the "disappearing positive methodology."[44] In this the first screening was done at the Moscow laboratory.

After the screening, the data with the name of the athlete would be sent to the Deputy Minister for Sport. A decision would be made whether to save the sample or quarantine the sample. In case the directive was to save, the Moscow laboratory would feed false data into the ADAMS, thereby allowing the athlete to compete. This would result in the lab reporting a positive analytical finding as a negative analytical finding.[45] This system however was not to be used in international events due to the presence of independent observers. Hence, for international competitions the Russian State developed the technique of switching samples. The FSB helped in opening supposedly tamper-proof bottles containing dirty samples. For Sochi, selected athletes were required to collect clean samples. Dr Rodchenko would test several of these to ensure that they were indeed clean.[46] Once an adequate quantity of clean samples was collected, the FSB would transport and store them in an FSB building, next to the accredited Sochi lab. The Sochi lab selected to conduct tests for the Sochi Games (both Winter Olympics and Paralympics) was to assist in sample swapping.[47] During the Games, the contaminated samples would be transported from the lab through a mouse hole. Dirty samples were passed from inside the secured premises to outside the secured premise. The B sample would be taken to an operation room where the clean sample, stored in the FEB freezer, would be exchanged. The dirty sample thus would be replaced. The clean urine would be filled in both A and B sample bottles. And then would be passed back into the secured premises of the lab through the mouse hole.[48]

Dr Rodchenko and the Ministry of Sport and FSB worked this brilliant scheme directly under the nose of WADA and the IOC. In fact, WADA and the IOC would not have had any knowledge but for Rodchenko's whistle-blowing. The sample-swapping technology was developed exclusively for the Sochi Games to evade the scrutiny of the international community. Once the Sochi Games were over, as per the IP report, Russia switched back to the disappearing-positive methodology.[49] Dr Rodchenko was also instrumental in the destruction of thousands of samples before the IC's visit as well as tampering with other dirty samples that

---

42 Ibid 10
43 Ibid 12
44 Ibid 10
45 Ibid 11
46 Ibid 13
47 Ibid (n 40) 14
48 Ibid
49 Ibid 15

could not be destroyed. Efforts were taken to ensure that the IC could not detect any evasion or manipulation.[50] On the whole, the IP report affirmed the finding of the IC regarding the complicity of the Moscow laboratory and RUSADA. The Sochi Games lab was only a small player in the doping cover-up. Importantly, however, the IP report came up with concrete findings about the involvement of the Russian Ministry of Sport in the doping scheme.[51] Interestingly, as per the IP report, the elaborate doping scheme with the help of disappearing-positive methodology was in operation since 2011. It was used to cover up doping in all sports. Further, 88 percent of the samples of foreign athletes tested by the Moscow lab were quarantined and reported as positive analytical findings, whereas, per the IP report, 89 percent of the samples of Russian athletes tested by the Moscow lab were saved and reported as negative analytical finding.[52]

Dr Rodchenko explained the sophisticated technique of ingesting the steroid he developed which prevented detection. Thus, Russian athletes could safely participate in the 2012 London Olympics without any detection. He fine-tuned the technique further, thus mastering the art of avoiding detection.[53] The IP observed that "[t]he picture that emerges from all of the foregoing is an intertwined network of State involvement through the MofS and the FSB in the operations of both the Moscow and Sochi Laboratories. The FSB was woven into the fabric of the Laboratory operations and the MofS was directing the operational results of the Laboratories."[54] The deep-rooted involvement of the Russian State and its manipulation of the anti-doping system challenges the legitimacy of the current system. As noted earlier, all the WADA-mandated standards and protocols were violated without fear. The question that needs to be asked is, what were the IOC and WADA doing? And if this is the case with Russia, one has to wonder which other countries might be manipulating the system. The advanced science and technology and the state power used in covering up and conning the Sochi Games points towards elitism. High-performing sports nations, with financial wherewithal, can rest easy because they can beat WADA at its own game. The IP report is a document of this power play.

As per the key findings of the IP report:

1. "The Moscow Laboratory operated, for the protection of doped Russian athletes, within a State-dictated failsafe system, described in the report as the Disappearing Positive Methodology."[55]
2. "The Sochi Laboratory operated a unique sample swapping methodology to enable doped Russian athletes to compete at the Games."[56]

50 Ibid 16–17
51 Ibid 35
52 Ibid 37–39
53 Ibid 49–51
54 Ibid 60
55 Ibid 86
56 Ibid

3   "The Ministry of Sport directed, controlled and oversaw the manipulation of athlete's analytical results or sample swapping, with the active participation and assistance of the FSB, Center of Sports Preparation of National Teams of Russia (CSP), and both Moscow and Sochi Laboratories."[57]

4   "The Moscow Laboratory personnel did not have a choice in whether to be involved in the State directed system."[58]

5   "The Moscow Laboratory operated under State directed oversight and control of its anti-doping operational system."[59]

6   "The Moscow Laboratory personnel were required to be part of the State directed system that enabled Russian athletes to compete while engaged in the use of doping substances."[60]

7   "The Moscow Laboratory was the final failsafe protective shield in the State directed doping regime."[61]

8   "Sample bottles stored in the Moscow Laboratory from 10 September to 10 December 2014 were tampered with by having their urine swapped."[62]

9   "The Disappearing Positive Methodology was planned and operated over a period from at least late 2011 until August 2015."[63]

10 "Russian athletes from the vast majority of summer and winter Olympic sports benefited from the Disappearing Positive Methodology."[64]

11 "The planning for the unique Sochi Laboratory sample swapping involved the Ministry of Sport, FSB, CSP, and the Moscow Laboratory." [65]

12 "A pre-selected group of Russian athletes competing at Sochi were protected by the Sochi sample swapping methodology."[66]

13 "Every sample bottle the IP investigation team examined revealed evidence of tampering consistent with the caps being removed and reused."[67]

14 "The Ministry of Sport made the determination as to which athletes would be protected by the Disappearing Positive Methodology."[68]

15 "The Deputy Minister of Sport in his discretion made the save or quarantine order."[69]

16 "Russian officials knew that Russian athletes competing at Sochi used doping substances."[70]

57 Ibid
58 Ibid 87
59 Ibid
60 Ibid
61 Ibid
62 Ibid
63 Ibid 88
64 Ibid
65 Ibid
66 Ibid
67 Ibid
68 Ibid 89
69 Ibid
70 Ibid

17   "The precise method used by the FSB to open the Sochi sample bottles is unknown."[71]

18   "The IP experts conclusively established that the caps can be removed and reused later."[72]

The above-quoted points reiterate the argument being made throughout that the WADA anti-doping system is ineffective unless there is the will to implement it the way it was envisaged. Importantly, the IOC has again failed to live up to the role it propagates viz. the overseer of doping-free sport. The IOC was slow to react to the impact of the Russian doping scandal. With Sochi being tainted, the IOC's position as the supreme governing body was under threat. WADA's response to the IC recommendations was to declare RUSADA as being non-compliant with the WADA Code. Accordingly, RUSADA was removed from the list of WADA-recognized National Anti-Doping Organizations (NADOs).[73] Thus, from 18 November 2015 onwards RUSADA remained non-compliant to the WADA Code.

The conditions were laid down by WADA to enable RUSADA to become Code compliant viz. bringing in structural reforms, independence of the agency from the Russian government and upholding strong anti-doping values.[74] RUSADA was to cooperate and coordinate with WADA for proving transparency in anti-doping programme enforcement. Despite dissensions amongst the members of the WADA Executive Committee, RUSADA was declared Code compliant on 20 September 2018.[75] This decision has received severe criticism considering that WADA Vice President Linda Hofstad Helleland opposed the reinstatement of RUSADA.[76] In addition, executive members of Oceania also opposed the move.[77] The criticism is based on the fact that Russia has been reluctant to accept the findings of McLaren's report and have resisted WADA's access to its labs. Access to data is now made a condition that RUSADA needs to comply with post-reinstatement and not pre-reinstatement.[78] WADA President

71 Ibid
72 Ibid
73 WADA, "WADA Publishes RUSADA Roadmap to Code Compliance" (2017) www.wada-ama.org/en/media/news/2017-08/wada-publishes-rusada-roadmap-to-code-compliance (accessed 4 December 2018)
74 WADA, "Rusada: Roadmap to Compliance" (2017) www.wada-ama.org/sites/default/files/2017-08-02_rusada_roadmaptocompliance_en.pdf (accessed 3 December 2018)
75 WADA, "WADA Executive Committee decides to Reinstate RUSADA Subject to Strict Conditions" (2018) www.wada-ama.org/en/media/news/2018-09/wada-executive-committee-decides-to-reinstate-rusada-subject-to-strict-conditions (accessed 3 December 2018)
76 Lawrence Ostlere, "Wada Reinstates Russian Anti-Doping Agency in Defiance of Worldwide Outcry Against Disgraced Body's Credibility" Independent (London, 20 September 2018) www.independent.co.uk/sport/wada-rusada-russian-anti-doping-agency-reinstated-a8547021.html (accessed 3 December 2018)
77 Ibid
78 Ibid

Craig Reedie defended the decision to reinstate RUSADA by insisting that Russia has acknowledged the existence of systematic doping. Further, as per Reedie, Russia is cooperating by giving access to independent experts.[79] These claims, as of now, appear unsubstantiated. Why WADA could not have waited until Russia admitted to state-sponsored doping remains a question. Further, Reedie's defense of WADA's decision appears to fall flat in view of the clear findings in McLaren's report.

WADA's decision is based on the requirement that RUSADA provide access to data so that athletes found guilty on re-analyses will be acted against. This is punishing the athletes and making an example of them. The real perpetrators, that is, the state officials, are not punished or are not required to prove their innocence. WADA should have insisted on proof of complete autonomy of the Russian sports authority and clear commitment of the Russian government to clean up the system. The second report McLaren submitted to WADA gave further details of the conspiracy carried out by the Russian State.[80] Hence WADA should have insisted on the acknowledgement of these findings as facts. Sadly, this confirms that anti-doping is more about political bargaining and less about fairness. WADA clearly is ready to use the athletes as scapegoats. Unfortunately, WADA's ambiguous stance towards the Russian government is matched by IOC's. The IOC's initial response to the scandal fell way short of expectations. The IOC refused to impose a blanket ban on Russian athletes in the light of the finding of the IC report. On the contrary, it left each individual International Federation to decide upon the fate of Russian athletes. This decision to play it safe was taken by IOC for the 2016 Rio Summer Olympics.[81] The IOC's ambivalence on the issue was further reflected when it issued a statement declaring that each sport was to "carry out an individual analysis of each Russian athlete's anti-doping record, taking into account only reliable, adequate international tests, and the specificities of the athlete's sport and its rules, in order to ensure a level playing field."[82]

Thus, while the IOC reversed the rule pertaining to presumption of innocence in the case of athletes, it did not reverse the same in the case of the Russian State. Further, the IOC convened Disciplinary Commissions only upon the submission of WADA reports. This reveals that for the IOC anti-doping is independent of its obligations to ensure good governance in sports. Considering that the allegations pertained to manipulation in the Sochi Olympics, the delay on the part of IOC

79 Andy Brown, "Reedie Again Defends WADA's Decision to Reinstate Rusada" *The Sports Integrity Initiative* (2018) www.sportsintegrityinitiative.com/reedie-again-defends-wadas-decision-to-rein state-rusada/ (accessed 3 December 2018)
80 Richard H. Mclaren, O.C. Independent Person, "The Independent Person 2nd Report" *WADA Investigation of Sochi Allegations* (2016) www.wada-ama.org/sites/default/files/resources/files/ mclaren_report_part_ii_2.pdf (accessed 4 December 2018)
81 Sean Ingle, "Russia's Athletes Escape Blanket IOC Ban for Rio Olympic Games" *The Guardian* (London, 24 July 2016) www.theguardian.com/sport/2016/jul/24/russia-team-escape-blanket-ban-ioc-rio-olympic-games (accessed 3 December 2018)
82 Ibid

was surprising. The IOC invoked its power under bylaw 59 and convened two Disciplinary Commissions on 19 July 2016.[83] The First Commission was headed by Samuel Schmid, the Second Commission was headed by Denis Oswald.[84] Before the Schmid Commission, Dr Rodchenkov deposed and revealed in detail all that had been noted by the McLaren report.[85] The Schmid report, however, does not accept the existence of any state-sponsored doping in Russia. It accepts the explanation given by the Russian government that it was more the fault of individuals than the Russian institutions.[86] The IOC Disciplinary Commission report thus completely diverges from the findings of the IC and the McLaren reports. The Schmid report primarily relies on the language used by McLaren in his second report vis-à-vis the key findings. As per the McLaren report, one of the key findings was that

> An institutional conspiracy existed across summer and winter sports athletes who participated with Russian officials within the Ministry of Sport and its infrastructure, such as the RUSADA, CSP and the Moscow Laboratory, along with the FSB for the purposes of manipulating doping controls. The summer and winter sports athletes were not acting individually but within an organised infrastructure as reported on in the 1st Report.[87]

Interestingly, the reference to an institutional conspiracy rather than a state-run conspiracy is seen as evidence of the lack of proof of state doping. What the Schmid report fails to note is that McLaren reaffirms in the final report the key findings of the first report. Amongst other findings, he reiterates that

> The Moscow Laboratory operated, for the protection of doped Russian athletes, within a State-dictated failsafe system, described in the report as the Disappearing Positive Methodology.[88]

This point is overlooked by the Schmid report, and thus the Russian State is let off the hook. The Schmid report does find that the Russian Olympic Committee (ROC) had breached its commitment to uphold the WADA Code.[89] Similarly, the Organizing Committee of the Olympic Winter Games Sochi 2014

83 IOC, "IOC Disciplinary Commission's Report to the IOC Executive Board" (2017) 4 https:// stillmed.olympic.org/media/Document%20Library/OlympicOrg/IOC/Who-We-Are/Commis sions/Disciplinary-Commission/IOC-DC-Schmid/IOC-Disciplinary-Commission-Schmid-Report.pdf (accessed 3 December 2018)

84 Ibid

85 Grigory M. Rodchenkov, "Affidavit of Dr. Grigory M. Rodchenkov" (2017) http://10ste93kec2 i6oi6nlhmxd19.wpengine.netdna-cdn.com/wp-content/uploads/2017/12/Schmid-Affidavit-GR-Text-Searchable-email.pdf (accessed 3 December 2018)

86 IOC (n 83) 24

87 Richard H. Mclaren (n 80) 1

88 Ibid 6

89 IOC (n 83) 26–27

(SOCOG) was held to be jointly and severally liable for the failures to imple-ment the WADA Code.[90] It holds the Russian Ministry of Sport liable for negli-gence to enforce the anti-doping rules,[91] though it does not find the Russian State guilty of state doping.

Following the Schmid Commission report, the IOC Executive Board took the decision to suspend the ROC but it permitted individual Russian athletes to compete in the 2018 Olympic Winter Games in Pyeongchang.[92] The participa-tion was to be based on an invitation list prepared by a committee as constituted by the IOC Executive Board. The Committee was composed of one representa-tive each from the Independent Testing Authority (ITA), Doping Free Sport Unit (DFSU), WADA and the IOC. The Russian athletes participated in the 2018 Winter Olympics under the designation "Olympic Athlete from Russia" (OAR).[93] It was this decision of the IOC which encouraged Russia to negotiate with WADA and convince it to reinstate RUSADA.[94] WADA represented the act of Russia accepting the IOC decision on the Winter Olympics as acceptance of Russia's guilt. Sir Craig Reedie failed to point out the fact that Russia agreed to provide access to data only under the supervision and control of its investigators. Russia did not make an unconditional commitment to cooperate. On the con-trary the indication is that Russia is dictating terms to WADA. Not surprisingly, Russia continues to maintain its official stand that the failure and fault lie with individuals, including athletes, thus it promises to cooperate with WADA to ini-tiate criminal prosecution against the guilty athletes.[95] At the end of this discus-sion we get a deep-rooted love for the powerful and the winners. WADA and the IOC have chosen to be ambivalent in dealing with the Russian doping scandal. Their stance on the role of the Russian State is proof of existing contradictions in the anti-doping narrative. At the moment, however, the policy appears to be see no evil, hear no evil and speak no evil. The developed, rich countries continue to rule with elitism and dominance.

The aftertaste – it's bitter! For all?

The decision of the IOC to permit selected Russian athletes to participate in the Olympic Winter Games PyeongChang 2018 led to challenges before

90 Ibid
91 Ibid 28
92 IOC, *Decision of the IOC Executive Board* (Lausanne, 2017) https://stillmed.olympic.org/media/Document%20Library/OlympicOrg/IOC/Who-We-Are/Commissions/Disciplinary-Commission/IOC-DC-Schmid/Decision-of-the-IOC-Executive-Board-05-12-2017.pdf (accessed 3 December 2018)
93 Ibid
94 Pavel Kolobkov's Letter to Sir Craig Reedie (2018) www.wada-ama.org/sites/default/files/20180913_letterfromrussianministry_to_wada.pdf (accessed 3 December 2018)
95 The Editorial Board, "The World Anti-Doping Agency Cleared Russia. Based on What?" *Opinion* (2018) www.nytimes.com/2018/09/25/opinion/editorials/russia-olympics-anti-doping.html (accessed 3 December 2018)

the Court of Arbitration for Sports (CAS). The background was the finding of the IOC Disciplinary Commission (IOC DC) chaired by Denis Oswald.[96] The terms of reference were re-analysis, including forensic analysis, and a full inquiry into all Russian athletes who participated in the 2014 Olympic Winter Games in Sochi as well as their coaches, officials and support staff.[97] The IOC DC imposed stringent sanctions on thirty-nine athletes. They were permanently barred from all editions of the Olympic Games. Of the several appeals filed before CAS, one is *Aleksandr Zubkov v. International Olympic Committee* (IOC).[98] Zubkov was one of the thirty-nine Russian athletes facing sanctions. Since they all appealed against the same decision of the IOC DC, the CAS collectively called them the "Sochi appellants." In this case the athletes collectively and individually challenged the sanctions by the IOC on several grounds. The first point was that the IOC misapplied the relevant legal framework.[99] It failed to assess individual cases of the athlete on their own merit. Rather, the IOC generalized the findings and applied a "'broad brush approach' to its assessment of the evidence."[100] The appellant challenged the presumption on the part of the IOC as to the existence of "an institutionalised system to protect certain doped athletes during the Sochi Games."[101] The athletes challenged the IOC's assumption that "particular individual athletes were involved in the scheme of institutionalised doping."[102] Accordingly, the appellant challenges the finding of the IOC that

> the individual Sochi Appellants must each have: (a) used the Duchess Cocktail; (b) provided clean urine to be used to replace dirty urine samples with clean ones; and (c) communicated the number of their doping control samples at the Sochi Games to the persons who were responsible for tampering with, and substituting the contents of, the samples provided by the Sochi Appellants during the doping control process.[103]

The appellants also challenged the inferences thus drawn by IOC in the absence of admissible evidence.

96 IOC, "Decision of the IOC Disciplinary Commission sitting in the Following Composition: Denis Oswald, Chairman Juan Antonio Samaranch, Tony Estanguet in the Proceedings Against Aleksandr Tretiakov" (2017) https://stillmed.olympic.org/media/Document%20Library/OlympicOrg/IOC/Who-We-Are/Commissions/Disciplinary-Commission/2017/SML-022-Decision-Disciplinary-Commission-Aleksandr-TRETIAKOV.pdf (accessed 3 December 2018)
97 Ibid 5
98 CAS 2017/A/5422
99 Ibid para 73
100 Ibid
101 Ibid
102 Ibid
103 Ibid

The IOC's finding on tampering of samples has also been challenged as being too general.[104] The athletes argued that they were denied the opportunity to counter the evidence relied upon by the IOC.[105] They challenged the credibility of Dr Rodchenkov as a witness.[106] Similarly, they challenged the credibility of other witnesses relied upon by the McLaren report.[107] Thus, they challenged the findings of an Anti-Doping Rule Violation (ADRV). They asserted that under the then-existing WADA Code there was no ground to conclude an ADRV on "a vague notion of conspiracy."[108] Further the IOC, as per the athletes, wrongly applied the concept of conspiracy and complicity to their cases,[109] thus there was no evidence to prove an ADRV. They also alleged that "the proceedings before the IOC DC violated their fundamental due process rights."[110] The athletes were not given hearing during the IOC investigations.[111] The IOC did not give them reasonable opportunity to peruse the materials relied upon by the IOC to arrive at its conclusion. As per the athletes, the IOC "'held back evidence until the /last possible moment' . . . with the result that the Sochi Appellants were unable to prepare their defences in an adequate manner." Further, as per the athletes, "the IOC refused, and in some instances continues to refuse, the Sochi Appellants' requests for access to relevant documents and evidence in the IOC's possession."[112] The athletes also argued that they did not get the opportunity to cross-examine Dr Rodchenkov or Prof McLaren. Thus, the athletes argue that the IOC:

(a) failed to disclose in a timely manner the evidence that would be used against them; (b) withheld key evidence and information; (c) failed to provide a proper opportunity for the Sochi Appellants to review reports and analyses; and (d) failed to provide the Sochi Appellants with a proper opportunity to file rebuttal evidence in response to the IOC's evidence.[113]

Accordingly, these acts of the IOC amounted to "'repeated breaches' of the Sochi Appellants' fundamental due process rights" and "impugn the legitimacy of the entire process and vitiate the validity of the IOC DC's decisions."[114]

The athletes argued that the burden of proof was on the IOC to establish "to the /comfortable satisfaction of the Panel, that the Sochi Appellants have committed

---

104 Ibid para 75
105 Ibid para 78–79
106 Ibid para 88
107 Ibid para 122
108 Ibid para 77
109 Ibid
110 CAS 2017/A/5422 (n 98) para 78
111 Ibid para 79
112 Ibid
113 Ibid para 80
114 Ibid para 81

ADRVs."[115] They proceeded on the premise that the evidence relied upon by the IOC was not strong enough to prove such grave allegations. The appellants challenged the IOC's finding that the athletes had violated Article 2.2, Article 2.5 and Article 2.8 of the 2009 WADA Code.[116] On the finding of an ADRV based on Article 2.5, they challenged the applicability of strict liability standards to the allegations of tampering. Their reasoning was that "It would be contrary to natural justice for an athlete to be found to have committed an ADRV in circumstances where an athlete provides a clean urine sample, which is then used without his/her knowledge by a third party in a process which the athlete has no knowledge of."[117] Further, they asserted "that the provision of clean urine alone does not fall under the Prohibited Method of urine substitution." They challenged the findings of an ADRV on the basis of Article 2.8 of the 2009 Code, arguing that

> [w]hereas "conspiracy" is expressly referred to in Article 2.9 of the 2015 WADC, "conspiracy" is not referred to in Article 2.8 of the 2009 WADC. Instead, under the 2009 WADC "conspiracy" is merely a possible aggravating circumstance pursuant to Article 10.6. It is not an independent ground for a finding of an ADRV. For the purposes of Article 2.8 of the WADC, complicity or cover-up requires proof that the athlete is acting with intent, i.e. with a degree of knowledge of the actions he/she is complicit in. Consequently, in order to establish a violation of Article 2.8 of the WADC against an individual athlete, the IOC must demonstrate not only that the athlete committed an act which assisted or covered up the commission of an ADRV by a third party, but that they did so with the intention of assisting or covering up that ADRV.[118]

Thus the finding of conspiracy was questionable, as per the athletes.

Dr Rodchenkov's credibility as a witness was challenged on the basis that his testimony was not verified by other witnesses or other documentary evidence.[119] Further, Dr Rodchenkov's statement needs to be considered in context. He was desperate to remain in the US; he was facing the threat of deportation to Russia with the prospect of criminal prosecution. Hence, as per the athletes, he needed to tell a spectacular story to implicate the Russian State. Hence, he was not a credible witness.[120] His intentions are not above board considering that he did not come clean before the IC.[121] He instead chose to hog the limelight by revealing the story to the media. The athletes portrayed Dr Rodchenkov as a publicity-seeking witness without any credibility. He was alleged to be inconsistent in the statements

115 Ibid para 83
116 Ibid para 85
117 Ibid para 86
118 Ibid para 87
119 Ibid para 89
120 Ibid para 90
121 Ibid para 91

that he was making.[122] Importantly, the athletes challenged Dr Rodchenkov's credibility by stating that he is a criminal and a drug dealer.[123] He was found by the IC "to be personally involved in the manipulation of blood and urine samples for his own financial gain, including by soliciting and accepting bribes. As such, he had a clear motive to blame his own wrongdoing on others."[124] Finally vis-à-vis Dr Rodchenkov, the appellants alleged that his statements based on his personal diary entries had no probative value.[125] The appellants further claimed that they had not tested positive for any PEDs; hence, there was no evidence against them of having committed an ADRV.[126] Further, there was no proof of them having switched their urine samples or given urine outside the routine procedures.[127]

They also argued that they never communicated with any third party conveying any information with respect to their samples.[128] They also dismissed the veracity of all indirect evidence, like scratch marks on sample bottles, high salt content and DNA analysis.[129] They argued that there was none to prove an ADRV. They also challenged the probative value of the witness testimony relied upon by Prof McLaren.[130] Thus the Sochi appellants also challenged the sanction imposed. Their argument was that even if there was proof of an ADRV, the sanctions imposed by the IOC were "grossly disproportionate."[131] The IOC DC banned the Sochi appellants from participation in "all editions of the Games of the Olympiad and the Olympic Winter Games subsequent to the Sochi Olympic Winter Games."[132] This was more than what the 2009 WADA Code prescribed.[133] Further, imposition of a life ban on athletes has to be based upon a proper analysis of each individual athlete's case. As per the appellants, "the IOC must have regard to the specific circumstances of each individual athlete's case and must provide proper reasons for its decision to impose the maximum sanction."[134] Since the IOC imposed blanket sanctions, it failed to consider their individual circumstances. Understandably, the IOC refuted each and every allegation made by the Sochi appellants. For instance, it insisted on the veracity of the indirect evidence viz. scratch marks, salt content and DNA analysis.[135] The IOC also affirmed the validity of Dr Rodchenkov's witness statement.[136] The IOC further affirmed that it met the requisite standard of burden of proof viz.

122 Ibid para 92
123 Ibid para 94
124 Ibid
125 Ibid para 95
126 Ibid para 97
127 Ibid para 98
128 Ibid para 99
129 Ibid para 100–121
130 Ibid para 122
131 Ibid para 124
132 IOC (n 96) 44
133 CAS 2017/A/5422 (n 98) para 125
134 Ibid para 129
135 Ibid para 165–174
136 Ibid para 175

comfortable satisfaction of the Panel, which is lower than proof beyond reasonable doubt and higher than balance of probability.[137]

The IOC argued that the purely circumstantial evidence was good enough to establish an ADRV.[138] The IOC justified the lack of additional witnesses or other evidence to prove the involvement of Sochi appellants, by the surrounding circumstance.[139] The IOC argued that under the given scenario anyone giving a statement was susceptible to death threats. To prove the point, the IOC cited the example of Dr Rodchenkov and Yuliya Stepanova and her husband Vitaly Stepanov, who are living in hiding.[140] Hence, as per the IOC, there was enough evidence to prove the ADRV of the Sochi appellants. Further the appellants were involved in the cover-up conspiracy and sample swapping. The IOC argued that "each of the Sochi Appellants must have been fully aware that they were being protected under the doping and cover-up scheme. Any alternative scenario in which the Sochi Appellants were not personally implicated in and/ or aware of the scheme is simply implausible."[141] Further, the IOC asserted that "the IOC DC carefully considered each Appellant's circumstances on a case-by-case basis before concluding that it was comfortably satisfied that the involvement of the individual Appellant in the scheme was established."[142] The IOC also asserted that there was proof of tampering, and to prove an ADRV under Article 2.2 of the WADA Code 2009 neither intent nor knowledge nor negligence is needed.[143] Similarly, the Sochi appellants were proven to have committed the "ADRV of use of a Prohibited Substance."[144] The IOC repeated the argument of conspiracy, terming it as vertical conspiracy and thus in violation of Article 2.8.[145] Based on CAS jurisprudence, "vertical conspiracy" is defined as an act by which "an athlete who, for his own interests, participates in a conspiracy involving other athletes," and thus "commits a violation of Article 2.8 of the WADC."[146]

As per the IOC, the Sochi appellants were involved in

(a) providing clean urine for storage in the urine bank; (b) photographing their DCFs and transmitting the images to Ms. Rodionova; and (c) deliberately failing to close their sample bottles by not turning the plastic lid to the maximum number of clicks. Further, the IOC submits that the Sochi Appellants' assistance was of a repeated nature.[147]

---

137 Ibid para 183
138 Ibid para 184
139 Ibid para 185–186
140 Ibid para 187
141 Ibid para 195
142 Ibid para 196
143 Ibid para 200
144 Ibid para 202
145 Ibid para 205
146 Ibid
147 Ibid para 207

The IOC also denied violation of any due process rights of the Sochi appellants. Importantly, the IOC argued that since the CAS has the power of hearing proceedings *de novo*, "any violation of procedural rights at first instance is cured by these proceedings before the CAS."[148] The IOC defended the imposition of lifetime ban on the grounds that the "Sochi Appellants' conduct has shocked the world at large and constitutes 'the most serious example of systemic cheating in the history of Olympic sport.'"[149] The CAS was thus required to evaluate and determine the guilt of the appellants and the proportionality of the IOC's decision. Accordingly, Dr Rodchenkov and Prof McLaren testified before the CAS panel. They both were cross-examined by the Sochi appellants.[150] Other witnesses also testified before the CAS panel, including IOC forensic expert Prof Christophe Champod.[151] He was countered by the Sochi appellants through the submission of Geoffrey Arnold, a senior consultant forensic scientist.[152] The Sochi appellants also relied upon the expert witness testimony of Alexey Bushin and Evgeniya Burova, who are both forensic experts and members of the Russian Federal Centre of Forensic Science.[153]

To prove the evidence gathered from DNA analysis, the IOC relied on the expert witness testimony of Dr Vincent Castella, the head of the Forensic Genetics Laboratory at the University Centre of Legal Medicine in Lausanne, Switzerland.[154] The Sochi appellants countered the IOC's submission on the veracity of DNA evidence by producing Dr Susan Pope, a Fellow of the Chartered Society of Forensic Scientists.[155] The IOC took the help of Prof Michael Burnier, the head of the Nephrology Service at University Hospital in Lausanne, Switzerland, for proving the claims based on salt content analysis.[156] The IOC was countered by the Sochi appellants through the expert witness of Dr David M. Charytan, an Assistant Professor of Medicine at Harvard Medical School, a qualified medical doctor and the Director of Intensive Care Nephrology at Brigham and Women's Hospital in Boston, Massachusetts.[157] Having thus heard both sides on all the points, the CAS gave its finding on each issue. The issue of jurisdiction was clearly ruled in favour of CAS, because R 47 of the CAS Code read with Article 11.2 of the IOC ADR for Sochi Games settled the matter.[158] The issue of limitation was also ruled in favour of the appellants, as the same was filed within the time limit of twenty-one days.[159] The IOC ADR for the Sochi Games was regarded as the applicable law, along with the Olympic Charter. In addition, the

148 Ibid para 210
149 Ibid para 214
150 Ibid para 268–330
151 Ibid para 389
152 Ibid para 442
153 Ibid para 454
154 Ibid para 473
155 Ibid para 484
156 Ibid para 499
157 Ibid para 544
158 Ibid para 641
159 Ibid para 649

2014 edition of the WADA Code list of prohibited substances was also regarded as the applicable law, as well as the WADA Code to the extent that the matter was not specifically covered by the IOC ADR.[160] The CAS accordingly referred to the 2009 WADA Code for the definition of an ADRV. The same was detailed in Articles 2.1 to 2.8. Further, the 2014 Prohibited List was relied upon for the definition of prohibited substances and prohibited methods.[161]

The burden and standard of proof were determined by CAS based on Article 3.1 of the WADA Code,[162] since the IOC ADR referred to the WADA Code for the same. Accordingly, the IOC had the burden of establishing that the Sochi appellants had committed an ADRV. The same was to be proven to the comfortable satisfaction of the Panel. Relying on its previous decisions, the CAS reiterated that it was a sliding scale, and hence the graver the offence the stricter the nature of proof needed to comfortably satisfy the Panel.[163] The CAS elaborated that

> [i]t is important to be clear, however, that the standard of proof itself is not a variable one. The standard remains constant, but inherent within that immutable standard is a requirement that the more serious the allegation, the more cogent the supporting evidence must be in order for the allegation to be found proven.[164]

Further, the CAS referred to Article 3.2 of the WADA Code to hold that

> all ADRVs except those involving the actual presence of a prohibited substance can be proven by "any reliable means" including, but not limited to, witness testimony and documentary. In addition, an ADRV under Article 2.2 of the WADC in the form of use or attempted use of a prohibited substance or prohibited method, may be established by reference to "other analytical information which does not otherwise satisfy all the requirements to establish" an ADRV based on presence of a prohibited substance.[165]

Having thus explained the concepts, the CAS went on to determine the extent to which the IOC had discharged its burden. Insisting that the standard of comfortable satisfaction is lesser than proof beyond reasonable doubt and greater than balance of probability, the CAS set about the task. The CAS declared that in determining an ADRV based on the said standard of proof, it would take into account all the relevant circumstances.[166]

For the present case, the CAS noticed the IOC's contention that the Sochi athletes were part of a conspiracy to cover up doping violations. Being secretive

---

160 Ibid para 650–655
161 Ibid
162 Ibid para 665
163 Ibid para 673
164 Ibid para 674
165 Ibid para 678
166 Ibid para 681–682

in nature, the IOC would not be in a position to produce direct evidence. Hence, the production of indirect evidence needed to be taken into account as substantiating claims of ADRV.[167] Further, the limitation on the nature of evidence procured by the IOC was due to the fact that it lacked investigatory powers like that of a state.[168] Thus, the IOC would use established facts to fill in the gaps that were the result of limited evidence.[169] However, the CAS insisted that

> it is insufficient for the IOC merely to establish the existence of an overarching doping scheme to the comfortable satisfaction of the Panel. Instead, the IOC must go further and establish, in each individual case, that the individual athlete knowingly engaged in particular conduct that involved the commission of a specific and identifiable ADRV. In other words, the Panel must be comfortably satisfied that the Athlete personally committed a specific violation of a specific provision of the WADC.[170]

Reliability of other types of evidence, documentary or non-documentary, would determine its acceptance by the Panel. The CAS panel clarified that the scope of its decision would be limited to only these appeals and was not a statement on the existence of large-scale doping in Russia and the Sochi Games.[171] The Panel also reiterated that being a *de novo* proceeding they were better situated than the IOC DC. The CAS had access to greater evidence and literature than the IOC DC.[172] Another important observation of the CAS was that

> The Panel does not consider it possible to conclude that the existence of a general doping and cover-up scheme automatically and inexorably leads to a conclusion that the Athlete committed the ADRVs alleged by the IOC. Instead, the Panel must carefully consider the ingredients of liability under each of the relevant provisions of the WADC that the Athlete is alleged to have contravened. It must then consider whether the totality of the evidence presented before the Panel enables it to conclude, to the requisite standard of comfortable satisfaction, that the Athlete personally committed the specific acts or omissions necessary to constitute an ADRV under each of those separate provisions of the WADC.[173]

The CAS thus proceeded to give its findings and decisions on each point. On swapping of urine samples, the CAS referred to Article 2.2 of the WADA Code

167 Ibid para 683
168 Ibid para 684
169 Ibid para 685
170 Ibid para 686
171 Ibid para 693
172 Ibid para 691–692
173 Ibid para 695

read with M2.1 of the 2014 Prohibited List.[174] The CAS concluded that for an ADRV under Article 2.2 read with M2.1, the athlete must personally swap the urine sample at the doping control station.[175] Since IOC did not allege swapping of urine samples by the Sochi appellants personally, it weakened the case of the IOC. The CAS reasoned that

> [t]he Panel does not consider, however, that this principle of strict liability applies in an identical fashion where the Athlete is alleged to have committed an act or omission that contributed to the substitution of the Athlete's urine by another person. Were it otherwise, then any athlete who provided a urine sample as part of normal doping control procedures would automatically commit an ADRV if a third party who is entirely unconnected with the athlete, and in respect of whom the athlete has no knowledge or control, later substitutes the content of the athlete's sample. Consequently, logic and fairness both dictate that strict liability under Article 2.2 of the WADC cannot automatically extend to everything that is done to an athlete's urine sample after he/she has provided it in accordance with a normal doping control procedure.[176]

Accordingly, the CAS held that an

> athlete who committed an act or omission that facilitated the later substitution of their own urine sample by the Sochi Laboratory will have committed an ADRV under Article 2.2 of the WADC if he/she committed the relevant act or omission with actual or constructive knowledge that their own urine sample was likely to be substituted.[177]

This meant that the intent or knowledge would matter where the swapping was done by a third party and not by the athlete personally.

This dilution of the strict liability rule in the given scenario further weakened the stance of the IOC. The IOC buttressed its claim by stating that (1) the appellants deliberately provided bottles of clean urine outside the doping control process, prior to the Sochi Games; (2) the appellants failed to close the bottles properly during the doping control test at the Sochi Games; and (3) the appellants transmitted the photos of the doping control forms to persons involved in sample swapping at the end of each doping control test.[178] The IOC used these arguments to prove the existence of knowledge. Unfortunately, on the first point the IOC could not produce any direct evidence, hence the same needed further corroboration.[179] The IOC referred to a list called the "Duchess List" that consisted

174 Ibid para 703
175 Ibid para 711
176 Ibid para 712
177 Ibid para 714
178 Ibid para 715
179 Ibid para 725

of the names of athletes who were to be given a cocktail of drugs. Unfortunately, not all of the Sochi appellants had their names on the list, and hence the list was not supportive of the IOC case.[180] Accordingly, as per the CAS,

> the Panel does not consider that the mere fact of the Athlete's presence on the Duchess List is sufficient in itself for the Panel to be comfortably satisfied that the Athlete used a prohibited substance during the Sochi Games, which would be indicative of the likely commission of the prohibited method of urine substitution.[181]

With regards to the second point, the IOC also had no direct evidence. On this, the CAS held that "*the Panel is unable to conclude to its comfortable satisfaction that the Athlete deliberately restricted the degree of closure of his sample bottles during the doping control process at the Sochi Games.*"[182] Similarly, with the third point there was no direct evidence. Again the CAS held that "*Having carefully considered the evidence presented by the Parties, and having regard to the absence of any direct evidence that the content of the Athlete's DCF was transmitted to any third party for this purpose, the Panel is unable to conclude to its comfortable satisfaction that the Athlete committed such an act or acts.*"[183]

The IOC came up with other arguments viz. (1) the presence of multiple T marks in the caps of the sample bottles; (2) highly elevated salt content as proof of bottle opening and (3) mixed DNA proof of bottle opening. On the first point the CAS concluded that

> the Panel, on the basis of the multiple T marks alone, is unable to conclude to the requisite comfortable satisfaction standard that the Athlete's sample bottles were in fact opened for the purpose of urine substitution. In addition, the Panel notes that marks on a bottle cannot themselves provide any direct evidence regarding the substances that were contained in the bottle when the marks were made. Finally, it has to be borne in mind that it has not been contended that the Athlete was personally involved in the actual physical reopening of any of his sample bottles.[184]

On the second point, however, the CAS went with the IOC's argument, concluding that the presence of abnormally high salt content was indicative of the fact that the urine sample had been swapped.[185] It also proved that the dirty sample was swapped with a clean urine sample. Further, access to a clean urine sample could only have been possible with the cooperation of the appellants. And the

180 Ibid para 728–732
181 Ibid para 735
182 Ibid para 745
183 Ibid para 751
184 Ibid para 760
185 Ibid para 777

appellants gave the clean urine with the knowledge that it would be used for urine sample swapping.[186] Accordingly, the CAS held that

> the Panel is comfortably satisfied both that: (a) the Athlete's urine samples from the Sochi Games were swapped with clean urine provided by the Athlete in advance of the Sochi Games; and (b) that the Athlete provided that clean urine in advance of the Sochi Games in the knowledge that it would be used for the purpose of carrying out unlawful urine substitution during the Sochi Games.[187]

The third point was dismissed as unsubstantiated.[188]

The Panel thus concluded, based on the evidence as provided by the IOC, that "the Athlete thereby committed an ADRV under Article 2.2 of the WADC in connection with M2.1 of the Prohibited List in the form of the use of a prohibited method."[189] The next point on which the Panel deliberated was whether there was use of a prohibited substance as per Article 2.2 of the WADA Code. For this, the IOC used the same evidence as set out above. The Panel arrived at similar conclusions. On the question of providing clean urine the Panel reiterated its finding that the appellants indeed provided the same.[190] On the Duchess List the conclusion was that the list was not enough to prove use of a prohibited substance.[191] However it might, along with other evidence, prove the same.[192] The Panel concluded that the deliberate faulty closure of the sample bottles was not evidence of use of a prohibited substance.[193] Alleged transmission of images of the doping control form was again dismissed as irrelevant or substantiated evidence.[194] The Panel also held that the presence of multiple T marks on the cap of the sample bottle did not prove an ADRV under Article 2.2.[195] However, elevated salt content was held to comfortably prove the use of prohibited substances under Article 2.1, as it proved the use of prohibited method under Article 2.2.[196] The argument based on mixed DNA was rejected.[197] The Panel went on to hold as its final conclusion that

> although the Panel does not consider that the mere presence of the Athlete's name on the Duchess List is in itself capable of establishing to the comfortable satisfaction of the Panel that the Athlete used the Duchess Cocktail, the

186 Ibid para 778–781
187 Ibid para 782
188 Ibid para 785
189 Ibid para 791
190 Ibid para 798
191 Ibid para 799
192 Ibid para 800
193 Ibid para 802
194 Ibid para 804
195 Ibid para 808
196 Ibid para 811
197 Ibid para 812

inclusion of the Athlete's name on the Duchess List is not entirely irrelevant when viewed in conjunction with the other evidence before the Panel. In particular, once it has been established that the Athlete deliberately facilitated the substitution of his urine by providing clean urine in advance of the Sochi Games, and that this course of conduct had a particular objective, i.e. to conceal his use of a prohibited substance, then it follows that the presence of the Athlete's name on the Duchess List provides some additional support for the conclusion that the Athlete did in fact use a prohibited substance, namely the prohibited substances which the Duchess Cocktail was composed of.[198]

Accordingly the ADRV under Article 2.2 was proven for the appellants involved in this case including Zubkov.

On the question of tampering of samples as under Article 2.5, the Panel noted that there was insufficient evidence as to the aspect of athletes doing things deliberately to tamper.[199] As explained above, there was insufficient proof to show that the athlete deliberately did not close the sample bottles.[200] Similarly, there was no sufficient proof to show that the pictures of doping control forms were transmitted to third parties by the athletes.[201] Hence, no ADRV was found under Article 2.5. Similarly, the Panel rejected the arguments of the IOC based on Article 2.8 by stating that

the Panel is not comfortably satisfied that the Athlete committed any act or omission that knowingly assisted, encouraged or covered up the commission of an ADRV under Article 2.2 to Article 2.7 of the WADC by any other athlete. Accordingly, the Panel does not find that the Athlete committed an ADRV under Article 2.8 of the WADC.[202]

Consequent to its analysis of the evidence the Panel went on to uphold the sanctions imposed by the IOC. The Panel supported its reasoning by citing the fact that with respect to the Olympics, the IOC alone has the jurisdiction to sanction. The same reasoning was provided within the IOC ADR for the Sochi Games.[203] However the Panel reduced the length of time for which the sanction was imposed. The IOC had sanctioned the athletes for all editions of Olympics. The Panel ruled against the same. As per the Panel, because there was no proof that the Sochi appellants participated in any cover-up of a larger sample-swapping scheme, the severity of the sanction was not proportional.[204] The Panel, unlike the IOC DC, was not convinced that the appellants were part of any conspiracy.

198 Ibid para 814
199 Ibid para 826
200 Ibid para 823
201 Ibid
202 Ibid para 849
203 Ibid para 877
204 Ibid para 883–884

Hence, the Panel held that "the Appellant is ineligible to compete in one edition of the Olympic Winer Games subsequent to the Sochi Games, i.e. the Olympic Winter Games 2018 in PyeongChang."[205]

The other case challenging the IOC's decision on the Sochi Games was *Alexander Legkov v. International Olympic Committee* (IOC).[206] In this case the IOC fared even worse. The Panel was not comfortably satisfied with any of the evidence produced by the IOC. The IOC relied on the same evidence as in the previous case. However, unlike the previous case where abnormal salt content saved the day, here there was no finding as to the presence of abnormal salt content in the athlete's sample. The IOC was not able to prove an ADRV under Article 2.2. As per the Panel,

> in order to be comfortably satisfied that the Athlete has committed an ADRV of use of a prohibited method, it is insufficient merely to establish the existence of a general sample-swapping scheme; rather, the Panel must be comfortably satisfied that the Athlete was personally and knowingly implicated in particular acts that formed part of, and facilitated the commission of, the substitution of his urine within that scheme. Since the Panel has come to the conclusion that, in the Athlete's case, none of the IOC's factual allegations have been proven to its comfortable satisfaction, the Panel concludes that it must reach the same conclusion regarding the Athlete's alleged use of a prohibited method as the Panel has reached in relation to his alleged use of a prohibited substance.[207]

Accordingly, the sanctions imposed on the athlete were overturned and he was free to participate in the Olympic Winter Games Pyeongchang 2018.

The CAS delivered similar decisions involving the Sochi appellants' cases. On the whole, of the thirty-nine cases appealed, the CAS found that in twenty-eight cases there was not sufficient proof of an ADRV. Accordingly, their appeal was upheld and sanctions were annulled and their results in the Sochi Games were retained. In the eleven cases the CAS upheld the decision of the IOC DC with one modification viz. the life ban was reversed. Thus, the ban was limited to only the Olympic Winter Games Pyeongchang 2018 and not to all of the Olympic editions. The IOC however did not invite the successful Sochi appellants to participate in the Olympic Winter Games Pyeongchang 2018. Accordingly, these appellants went for another round of arbitration before the CAS Ad Hoc Division formed for the 2018 Olympic Winter Games in Pyeongchang. The CAS Ad Hoc Division ruled that it did not have jurisdiction in these matters. The ruling was given on the technical grounds that the decision of the IOC to not invite was communicated well outside the ten-day limitation period. The Ad Hoc Division

205 Ibid para 886
206 CAS 2017/A/5379
207 Ibid para 827–828

could only hear matters that arose within a period of ten days prior to the start of the Olympics, hence this outcome appears obvious.[208] Further, the Ad Hoc Division also noted that the decision not to invite the successful Sochi appellants to the Olympic Winter Games Pyeongchang 2018 was not a sanction imposed by the IOC. Finally the Ad Hoc Division held that the IOC did not discriminate in preparing the invitation list for the OAR.[209] The aftereffects of the Sochi saga and Russian doping scandal thus continue to haunt many. However, it is the athletes who appear to have suffered and been victimized. This leaves a trail of uncertainty for those impacted. Importantly, from a developing country perspective, the scandal has left a bitter aftertaste.

Conclusion

What WADA did on 20 September 2018 was an encore of the IOC's performance on 28 February 2018.[210] On that day the IOC lifted the ban on the Russian Olympic Committee.[211] This was in compliance with the decision of the IOC Executive Board taken on 25 February 2018.[212] The IOC's laxity towards Russia is evident from the fact that during the Olympic Winter Games Pyeongchang 2018 two

208 Court of Arbitration for Sport, "Arbitration Rules for the Olympic Games" [Article 1 "Application of the Present Rules and Jurisdiction of the Court of Arbitration for Sport (CAS) The purpose of the present Rules is to provide, in the interests of the athletes and of sport, for the resolution by arbitration of any disputes covered by Rule 61 of the Olympic Charter, insofar as they arise during the Olympic Games or during a period of ten days preceding the Opening Ceremony of the Olympic Games. In the case of a request for arbitration against a decision pronounced by the IOC, an NOC, an International Federation or an Organising Committee for the Olympic Games, the claimant must, before filing such request, have exhausted all the internal remedies available to her/him pursuant to the statutes or regulations of the sports body concerned, unless the time needed to exhaust the internal remedies would make the appeal to the CAS Ad Hoc Division ineffective."] www.tas-cas.org/fileadmin/user_upload/CAS_Arbitration_Rules_Olympic_Games__EN_.pdf (accessed 4 December 2018)
209 For details see CAS OG 18/05 Pavel Abratkiewicz, Victor Sivkov, Anna Vychik, Evgeny Zykov, Anatoly Chelyshev, Danil Chaban, Konstantin Poltavets v. International Olympic Committee; CAS OG 18/02 Victor An, Vladimir Grigorev, Anton Shipulin, Evgeniy Garanichev, Ruslan Murashov, Ekaterina Shikhova, Sergei Ustyugov, Ksenia Stolbova, Ekaterina Urlova-Percht, Maksim Tcvetkov, Irina Uslugina, Yulia Shokshueva, Daria Virolainen, Dmitri Popo; CAS OG 18/03 Alexander Legkov, Maxim Vylegzhanin, Evgeniy Belov, Alexander Bessmertnykh, Evgenia Shapovalova, Natalia Matveeva, Aleksandr Tretiakov, Elena Nikitina, Maria Orlova, Olga Fatkulina, Alexander Rumyantsev, Artem Kuznetcov, Tatyana Ivanova, Albe; CAS OG 18/04 Tatyana Borodulina, Pavel Kulizhnikov, Alexander Loginov, Irina Starykh, Dimitry Vassiliev, Denis Yuskov v. International Olympic Committee
210 Martha Kelner, "Russia's Olympic Membership Restored by IOC After Doping Ban" The Guardian (London, 28 February 2018) www.theguardian.com/sport/2018/feb/28/russia-says-ioc-reinstated-membership-after-doping-allegations (accessed 5 December 2018)
211 IOC News, "IOC Statement" (2018) www.olympic.org/news/ioc-statement-2018-02-28 (accessed 5 December 2018)
212 IOC News, "Decision of the IOC Executive Board" (2018) www.olympic.org/news/decision-of-the-ioc-executive-board-2018-02-25 (accessed 5 December 2018)

athletes of the OAR tested positive for doping. Despite such infractions, the IOC lifted the ban on the ROC. The maximum punishment it imposed on the ROC for positive doping was to ban the athletes from the Closing Ceremony of the Olympic Winter Games PyeongChang 2018.[213] Thus two of the leading flag-bearers of anti-doping enforcement viz. WADA and IOC have welcomed back Russia. The other powerful International Sports Federation, the Fédération Internationale de Football Association (FIFA), has been equally accommodating towards Russia. FIFA ignored the hue and cry over Russian doping scandals and went along with the 2018 FIFA World Cup in Russia.[214] In this scenario, the power of the Russian State seems to overwhelm any will to deal with the issue of State doping. Further, as the CAS decisions reveal, the IOC's handling of the Russian doping cases was clumsy to say the least. Given the realities of such blatant favouritism towards a powerful elite sports nation, one really has no hope for the developing country athletes. This also sends a message that the powerful and rich can get away with breaking the rules. The latest series of controversies, post the Russian scandal, affirms this concern.[215] As will be seen in Chapter 4, the troika of WADA, the IOC and the International Federations are working hard to preserve the hegemony of the star athletes, the powerful nations and commercial corporate interests. On 4 December 2018, the IAAF decided not to reinstate Russian Athletics (RusAF).[216] The IAAF has set two conditions for the reinstatement of RusAF:

1   That the IAAF be given access to "all of the data and access to the samples that it needs to determine which of the Russian athletes in the LIMS database have a case to answer for breach of the IAAF anti-doping rules. The IAAF Council was clear that Russian athletes cannot return to international competition unconditionally until that issue is resolved one way or the other."[217]
2   That RusAF must pay for all the costs "incurred in the work of the Taskforce and in bringing or defending Russian cases at CAS. The IAAF Council was clear that this debt must be settled for reinstatement to occur; it is not fair to ask the IAAF and its other members to continue to carry these costs."[218]

213 Ibid
214 See 2018 FIFA World Cup Russia™-14 June–15 July www.fifa.com/worldcup/ (accessed 3 December 2018)
215 Shane Stokes, "Opinion: Why WADA and the UCI's Handling of the Froome Case Is Damaging to Sport" *CyclingTips* (2018) https://cyclingtips.com/2018/07/opinion-why-wada-and-the-ucis-handling-of-the-froome-case-is-damaging-to-sport/ (accessed 3 December 2018)
216 Associated Press, "'This Debt Must be Settled': IAAF Extends Russia's Doping Ban" *The Guardian* (London, 4 December 2018) www.theguardian.com/sport/2018/dec/04/iaaf-extends-russia-ban-athletics-debt-settled (accessed 5 December 2018)
217 IAAF Press Release, "IAAF Council Makes Key Decisions in Monaco" (Monaco, 2018) www.iaaf.org/news/press-release/budapest-awarded-2023-iaaf-world-championship (accessed 5 December 2018)
218 Ibid

Can the IAAF decision be regarded as a beacon of hope? Or is it a PR gimmick to bolster the image of the IAAF? One will await the effect, but there is a sense that such a one-off approach does not augur well for the world of sports. Consequentially, the stringent provision within the WADA Code appears to be meant to promote the interests of elite athletes and their nations. The next chapter looks at some of these provisions within the WADA Code to verify this concern.

Bibliography

Associated Press, "'This Debt Must Be Settled': IAAF Extends Russia's Doping Ban" *The Guardian* (London, 4 December 2018) www.theguardian.com/sport/2018/dec/04/iaaf-extends-russia-ban-athletics-debt-settled (accessed 5 December 2018)

Brown, Andy, "Reedie again defends WADA's decision to reinstate RUSADA" *The Sports Integrity Initiative* (2018) www.sportsintegrityinitiative.com/reedie-again-defends-wadas-decision-to-reinstate-rusada/ (accessed 3 December 2018)

CAS 2017/A/5379

CAS 2017/A/5422

CAS OG 18/02 Victor An, Vladimir Grigorev, Anton Shipulin, Evgeniy Garanichev, Ruslan Murashov, Ekaterina Shikhova, Sergei Ustyugov, Ksenia Stolbova, Ekaterina Urlova-Percht, Maksim Tcvetkov, Irina Uslugina, Yulia Shokshueva, Daria Virolainen, Dmitri Popo

CAS OG 18/03 Alexander Legkov, Maxim Vylegzhanin, Evgeniy Belov, Alexander Bessmertnykh, Evgenia Shapovalova, Natalia Matveeva, Aleksandr Tretiakov, Elena Nikitina, Maria Orlova, Olga Fatkulina, Alexander Rumyantsev, Artem Kuznetcov, Tatyana Ivanova, Albe

CAS OG 18/04 Tatyana Borodulina, Pavel Kulizhnikov, Alexander Loginov, Irina Starykh, Dimitry Vassiliev, Denis Yuskov v. International Olympic Committee

CAS OG 18/05 Pavel Abratkiewicz, Victor Sivkov, Anna Vychik, Evgeny Zykov, Anatoly Chelyshev, Danil Chaban, Konstantin Poltavets v. International Olympic Committee

Court of Arbitration for Sport, "Arbitration Rules for the Olympic Games" www.tas-cas.org/fileadmin/user_upload/CAS_Arbitration_Rules_Olympic_Games__EN_.pdf (accessed 4 December 2018)

The Editorial Board, "The World Anti-Doping Agency Cleared Russia. Based on What?" *Opinion* (2018) www.nytimes.com/2018/09/25/opinion/editorials/russia-olympics-anti-doping.html (accessed 3 December 2018)

IAAF Press Release, "IAAF Council Makes Key Decisions in Monaco" (Monaco, 2018) www.iaaf.org/news/press-release/budapest-awarded-2023-iaaf-world-championship (accessed 5 December 2018)

Ingle, Sean, "Russia's Athletes Escape Blanket IOC Ban for Rio Olympic Games" *The Guardian* (London, 24 July 2016) www.theguardian.com/sport/2016/jul/24/russia-team-escape-blanket-ban-ioc-rio-olympic-games (accessed 3 December 2018)

IOC, "Decision of the IOC Disciplinary Commission sitting in the Following Composition: Denis Oswald, Chairman Juan Antonio Samaranch, Tony Estanguet in the proceedings against Aleksandr Tretiakov" (2017) https://stillmed.olympic.org/media/Document%20Library/OlympicOrg/IOC/Who-We-Are/Commissions/Disciplinary-Commission/2017/SML-022-Decision-Disciplinary-Commission-Aleksandr-TRETIAKOV.pdf (accessed 3 December 2018)

IOC, "Decision of the IOC Executive Board" (Lausanne, 2017) https://stillmed.olympic.org/media/Document%20Library/OlympicOrg/IOC/Who-We-Are/Commissions/Disciplinary-Commission/IOC-DC-Schmid/Decision-of-the-IOC-Executive-Board-05-12-2017.pdf (accessed 3 December 2018)

IOC, "IOC Disciplinary Commission's Report to the IOC Executive Board" (2017) 4 https://stillmed.olympic.org/media/Document%20Library/OlympicOrg/IOC/Who-We-Are/Commissions/Disciplinary-Commission/IOC-DC-Schmid/IOC-Disciplinary-Commission-Schmid-Report.pdf (accessed 3 December 2018)

IOC News, "Decision of the IOC Executive Board" (2018) www.olympic.org/news/decision-of-the-ioc-executive-board-2018-02-25 (accessed 5 December 2018)

IOC News, "IOC Statement" (2018) www.olympic.org/news/ioc-statement-2018-02-28 (accessed 5 December 2018)

Kelner, Martha, "Russia's Olympic Membership Restored by IOC After Doping Ban" *The Guardian* (London, 28 February 2018) www.theguardian.com/sport/2018/feb/28/russia-says-ioc-reinstated-membership-after-doping-allegations (accessed 5 December 2018)

Mclaren, Richard H. O. C. Independent Person, "The Independent Person Report" *WADA Investigation of Sochi Allegations* (2016) www.wada-ama.org/sites/default/files/resources/files/20160718_ip_report_newfinal.pdf (accessed 3 December 2018)

Mclaren, Richard H. O. C. Independent Person, "The Independent Person 2nd Report" *WADA Investigation of Sochi Allegations* (2016) www.wada-ama.org/sites/default/files/resources/files/mclaren_report_part_ii_2.pdf (accessed 4 December 2018)

Ostlere, Lawrence, "Wada Reinstates Russian Anti-doping Agency in Defiance of Worldwide Outcry Against Disgraced Body's Credibility" *Independent* (London, 20 September 2018) www.independent.co.uk/sport/wada-rusada-russian-anti-doping-agency-reinstated-a8547021.html (accessed 3 December 2018)

Pavel Kolobkov's Letter to Sir Craig Reedie (2018) www.wada-ama.org/sites/default/files/20180913_letterfromrussianministry_to_wada.pdf (accessed 3 December 2018)

Pells, Eddie, "60 Minutes: WADA Received 200 Emails from Whistleblower About Russian Doping Scandal" *The Associated Press* (New York, 9 May 2016) www.cbc.ca/sports/olympics/russia-doping-scandal-whistleblower-1.3572938 (accessed 2 December 2018)

Prospero, '"Icarus' Reveals the Mastermind Behind Russia's Doping Programme" *The Economist* (London, 8 August 2017) www.economist.com/prospero/2017/08/08/icarus-reveals-the-mastermind-behind-russias-doping-programme (accessed 2 December 2018)

Rodchenkov, Grigory M. "Affidavit of Dr. Grigory M. Rodchenkov" (2017) http://10ste93kec2i6oi6nlhmxd19.wpengine.netdna-cdn.com/wp-content/uploads/2017/12/Schmid-Affidavit-GR-Text-Searchable-email.pdf (accessed 3 December 2018)

Ruiz, Rebecca R. and Michael Schwirtz, "Russian Insider Says State-Run Doping Fueled Olympic Gold" *The New York Times* (New York, 12 May 2016) www.nytimes.com/2016/05/13/sports/russia-doping-sochi-olympics-2014.html (accessed 3 December 2018)

Smith, R. Cory, "Olympic Medal Count 2014: Final Standings and Sochi Medal Tally for Each Country" *Bleacher Report* (2014) https://bleacherreport.com/articles/1970880-olympic-medal-count-2014-final-standings-and-sochi-medal-tally-for-each-country (accessed 2 December 2018)

Stokes, Shane, "Opinion: Why WADA and the UCI's Handling of the Froome Case Is Damaging to Sport" *CyclingTips* (2018) https://cyclingtips.com/2018/07/opinion-why-wada-and-the-ucis-handling-of-the-froome-case-is-damaging-to-sport/ (accessed 3 December 2018)

Tennis, Lucky Loser, "H. Seppelt – The Secrets of Doping – the Shadowy World of Athletics – ARD 2015 – English" *You Tube* (2015) www.youtube.com/watch?v=nIkiC3iT0GA (accessed 2 December 2018)

Tennis, Lucky Loser, "The Secrets of Doping: How Russia Makes Its Winners – H. Seppelt (ARD – 2014)" *YouTube* (2015) www.youtube.com/watch?v=iu9B-ty9JCY&t=7s (accessed 2 December 2018)

2018 FIFA World Cup Russia™-14 June–15 July www.fifa.com/worldcup/ (accessed 3 December 2018)

WADA, "Independent Commission-Terms of Reference" (2015) www.wada-ama.org/sites/default/files/wadaindependent-commission-terms-of-reference-2015-jan-en.pdf (accessed 3 December 2018)

WADA, "Independent Commission Terms of Reference (Addendum)" (2015) www.wada-ama.org/sites/default/files/resources/files/wada-independent-commission-tor-addendum-en.pdf (accessed 3 December 2018)

WADA, "Independent Investigation into the Sochi Allegations made by Grigory Rodchenkov" (2016) www.wada-ama.org/sites/default/files/resources/files/wada-independent-investigation-of-g-rodchenkov-allegations-tor-en_0.pdf (accessed 4 December 2018)

WADA, "Rusada: Roadmap to Compliance" (2017) www.wada-ama.org/sites/default/files/2017-08-02_rusada_roadmaptocompliance_en.pdf (accessed 3 December 2018)

WADA, "Statement regarding Extended Mandate of Independent Commission" (2015) www.wada-ama.org/en/media/news/2015-08/statement-regarding-extended-mandate-of-independent-commission (accessed 3 December 2018)

WADA, "WADA announces details of Independent Commission" (2014) www.wada-ama.org/en/media/news/2014-12/wada-announces-details-of-independent-commission (accessed 3 December 2018)

WADA, "WADA Executive Committee Decides to Reinstate RUSADA Subject to Strict Conditions" (2018) www.wada-ama.org/en/media/news/2018-09/wada-executive-committee-decides-to-reinstate-rusada-subject-to-strict-conditions (accessed 3 December 2018)

WADA, "WADA Publishes RUSADA Roadmap to Code Compliance" (2017) www.wada-ama.org/en/media/news/2017-08/wada-publishes-rusada-roadmap-to-code-compliance (accessed 4 December 2018)

WADA Code 2015, "Fundamental Rationale for the World Anti-Doping Code" www.wada-ama.org/sites/default/files/resources/files/wada-2015-world-anti-doping-code.pdf (accessed 3 December 2018)

WADA Independent Commission, "The Independent Commission Report #1 Final Report" *The Independent Investigation* (2015) www.wada-ama.org/sites/default/files/resources/files/wada_independent_commission_report_1_en.pdf (accessed 3 December 2018)

WADA Independent Commission, "The Independent Commission Report #2" *Independent Commission Investigation* (2016) www.wada-ama.org/sites/default/files/resources/files/wada_independent_commission_report_2_2016_en_rev.pdf (accessed 3 December 2018)

Yuan, Jada, "How Bryan Fogel Accidentally Documented the Russian Olympic Doping Scandal-And helped its key player escape to the United States" *Vulture* (2017) www.vulture.com/2017/12/icarus-bryan-fogel-russia-doping-scandal-olympics-netflix.html (accessed 3 December 2018)

Chapter 3

Relook at the WADA Code

An elitist paradigm or an inclusive document?

Introduction

This chapter carries the discussion forward, from where the previous chapter ends, dealing with issues that are perceived to affect both the rights of athletes as well as effective implementation of the WADA Code. The first issue that will be highlighted in this chapter is the strict liability doctrine. This doctrine imposes a one-size-fits-all approach on anti-doping regulations. The effect of this doctrine on the rights of athletes is a matter of concern. More so if the same relates to an athlete from a developing country/non-elite athlete. Associated with this issue is the burden of proof placed on the athlete and governing bodies. The problem that lack of intent creates at the stage of Adverse Analytical Finding/Adverse Non-Analytical Finding, is equally the result of adopting strict liability doctrine. There are justifications for this doctrine but the counterarguments are also strong enough to be taken note of. The other concern is the therapeutic use exemption granted under the WADA Code. The justification of granting such an exemption is spelled out in the Code and its regulations, but its use by elite athletes has been a matter of debate. It therefore needs to be analysed as to whether the said guidelines affirm to the stated objectives of the WADA Code. The final issue that will be touched upon by this chapter is the controversy on decision limits under WADA. On the whole, however, the viewpoint that this chapter tries to uphold is an inclusive approach, as against the elitist approach that the existing rules try to favour.

Strict liability and doping – a rough ride for the non-elite sportsperson

In USA Shooting & Q./Union Internationale de Tir (UIT),[1] the CAS said that "in principle the high objectives and practical necessities of the fight against doping amply justify the application of a strict liability standard."[2] This statement encapsulates the current philosophy governing the WADA Code. The strict liability principle proceeds on the assumption that all are guilty unless proven

---

1 CAS 94/129
2 Ibid para 16

innocent. In the UIT case[3] the CAS expressed concern that in the absence of a strict liability rule, sports federations would not be able to prove doping against athletes. The CAS strongly felt that "a requirement of intent would invite costly litigation that may well cripple federations-particularly those run on modest budgets-in their fight against doping."[4] The most telling statement of the CAS in the UIT case[5] was that unfairness to one individual does not necessarily make strict liability problematic as a principle. The interest of the larger community needs to be balanced against an individual's interest. As per the CAS, "it appears to be a laudable policy objective not to repair an accidental unfairness to an individual by creating an intentional unfairness to the whole body of other competitors."[6] The essence of this argument is the concept of a level playing field. Using performance-enhancing substances is said to tip the competitive edge in favour of the user against the rest. The CAS rejected all concerns pertaining to the unreasonableness of the strict liability principle or that it was "contrary to natural justice, because it does not permit the accused to establish moral innocence."[7] The CAS also rejected the argument that the strict liability principle "is an excessive restraint of trade."[8]

Justifications for strict liability have been given by others on more or less similar lines.[9] Toit argues that "In cases such as anti-doping rule violations it will be very difficult if not impossible to proof that the defendant had acted with fault or negligence."[10] In *Gasser v. Stinson & Another*,[11] J. Scott justified it by declaring that if an athlete or their support staff denied doping, it would be next to impossible for the Federation to disprove the claim. The requirement of intent would, as per J. Scott, render the anti-doping programme redundant. Summing up the justification for strict liability, J. Scott opined that "if a defence of moral innocence were open, the floodgates would be opened and the [Sport Governing Body's] attempts to prevent drug-taking by athletes would be rendered futile." This statement is no different from the position that the CAS took in UIT.[12] The whole point is the impossibility of proving "moral innocence." At present, there is no plan of abandoning the rule; on the contrary, it will continue to be

3 Ibid
4 Ibid para 15
5 Ibid
6 Ibid
7 Ibid para 16
8 Ibid
9 Thomas Wyatt Cox, "The International War Against Doping: Limiting the Collateral Damage from Strict Liability" (2014) *Vanderbilt Journal of Transnational Law*, 47 www.vanderbilt.edu/wp-content/uploads/sites/78/CoxFinalReviewComplete.pdf (accessed 23 April 2017)
10 Niel du Toit, "Strict Liability and Sports Doping – What Constitutes a Doping Violations and What Is the Effect Thereof on the Team?" (2011) *International Sports Law Journal*, 163 www.doping.nl/media/kb/2044/20131023T040659-ISLJ_2011_3-4%20-%20163-164%20Niel%20du%20Toit.pdf (accessed 22 April 2017)
11 Queens Bench Division, *Lexis Nexis Academic* (Transcript, Blackwell & Partners, 1988)
12 Arbitration CAS 94/129 (n 1)

the underlying doctrine for all future anti-doping rule violations. Sebastian Coe, writing for *The Telegraph*, emphatically stated that "strict liability – under which athletes have to be solely and legally responsible for what they consume – must remain supreme . . . we cannot, without blinding reason and cause, move one millimeter from strict liability – if we do, the battle to save sport is lost."[13] Sebastian Coe is currently the president of the IAAF. Thus, the place of strict liability is secure with overwhelming support for the principle.

From a non-elite athlete's perspective, the counterarguments to strict liability make sense. The unreasonableness and scope of injustice are greater in the case of a non-elite developing country athlete. McCutcheon gives the following instances of potential injustices that are likely to occur due to the application of the strict liability principle:

> the athlete's condition might be the result of any number of circumstances that do not involve fault on his or her part: a prescription error by a medical advisor, a dispensing error by a pharmacist, an honest and reasonable belief that the substance was not prohibited or the malicious act of a third party.[14]

In the developing country context, the aforementioned situations have the chance of occurring with greater frequency, as will be discussed in the subsequent chapter. In the non-elite context, each of these situations would be problematic in terms of evidence and burden of proof. Rebutting the findings of an ADRV itself means challenging the result management process. Importantly, it is for the athlete to debunk the cause of action that the federation relies upon to prove an ADRV. It requires taking on the might of the federation and overcoming the constraints imposed by unequal bargaining power. Evidently these are unrealistic expectations considering the circumstances of a non-elite developing country athlete. Cox rightly notes that

> [strict liability] seems an unfair approach given that guilt (which in the context implies that the person is a cheat) as a concept is morally loaded. Moreover, given that it essentially permits an innocent athlete to be deprived of his or her livelihood (and indeed possibly to have his or her career terminated) it is highly questionable.[15]

This statement and other arguments given against the application of strict liability echoes the fear and the vulnerabilities of a non-elite athlete.

13 Sebastian Coe, "We Cannot Move from Strict Liability Rule" *The Telegraph* (London, 5 February 2004) www.telegraph.co.uk/sport/othersports/drugsinsport/2373729/We-cannot-move-from-strict-liability-rule.html
14 Paul McCutcheon, "Sports Discipline, Natural Justice and Strict Liability" (1999) 28 *Anglo-American Law Review* 37
15 Neville Cox, "Legalisation of Drug use in Sport" (2002) 2 *ISLR* 77

WADA Code and strict liability – softening the rigour?

The above discussion on the justifications for and the fear against the strict liability principle notwithstanding, the same has been integrated into the WADA Code. Article 2.1.1 of the WADA Code states that

> it is each athlete's personal duty to ensure that no Prohibited Substance enters his or her body. Athletes are responsible for any Prohibited Substance or its Metabolites or Markers found to be present in their Samples. Accordingly, it is not necessary that intent, fault, negligence or knowing use on the athlete's part be demonstrated in order to establish an anti-doping rule violation.[16]

The comment to Article 2.1.1 also reiterates that an ADRV under this article is proven in disregard of athlete's fault/intent.[17] Further, Appendix 1 of the WADA Code defines strict liability as "[t]he rule which provides that . . . it is not necessary that intent, fault, negligence, or knowing use on the athlete's part be demonstrated by the anti-doping organization in order to establish an anti-doping rule violation."[18] Article 2.2.1 of the WADA Code also uses the strict liability principle for ADRVs.[19] The presumption of knowledge in strict liability, as stated above, does away with the requirement of fault. The only thing that matters is the act of enhancing sporting performance.[20] The principle focuses more on the act than the intention and affects personal liberty and autonomy.

It needs to be noted that the origins of strict liability as an acceptable principle of law have been justified on the basis of protecting harm to others. Importantly, it aimed at making defendants liable in situations where public safety or health were at stake or public interest was involved.[21] Viewed from this perspective, there is no specific justification, given within the WADA Code for adopting the strict liability principle. Understandably the basis is the UIT case which emphatically recognized the strict liability principle as the only way to tackle doping in sports.[22] As per Article 2, in addition to the presence or use

16 World Anti-Doping Agency, "World Anti-Doping Code" (2015) www.wada-ama.org/sites/default/files/resources/files/wada-2015-world-anti-doping-code.pdf (accessed 27 April 2017)
17 Ibid
18 Ibid 141
19 World Anti-Doping Agency (n 16) [it is each athlete's personal duty to ensure that no Prohibited Substance enters his or her body and that no Prohibited Method is used. Accordingly, it is not necessary that intent, fault, negligence or knowing use on the athlete's part be demonstrated in order to establish an anti-doping rule violation for use of a Prohibited Substance or a Prohibited Method]
20 J. R. Spencer, "Strict Liability and the European Convention" (2004) 63 (1) *Cambridge Law' Journal* 10
21 Ben Fitzpatrick, "Strict Liability: Importation Offence" (2004) 68 (3) *Journal of Criminal Law* 195
22 Jack Anderson, *Modern Sports Law-a Textbook* (Hart Publishing, 2010)

of prohibited substance or method, anti-doping rule violation is constituted when:

1   There is proof of athlete evading, refusing or failing to submit to sample collection.[23]
2   There are whereabouts failures.[24]
3   There is tampering or attempted tampering with any part of doping control.[25]
4   There is possession of a prohibited substance or a prohibited method.[26]
5   There is trafficking or attempted trafficking in any prohibited substance or prohibited method.[27]
6   There is administration or attempted administration to any athlete in-competition of any prohibited substance or prohibited method, or administration or attempted administration to any athlete out-of-competition of any prohibited substance or any prohibited Method that is prohibited out-of-competition.[28]
7   There is assisting, encouraging, aiding, abetting, conspiring, covering up or any other type of intentional complicity involving an anti-doping rule violation, attempted anti-doping rule violation or violation of Article 10.12.1 by another Person.[29]
8   There is prohibited association.[30]

Though "attempted use" of prohibited substance or method under Article 2.2.2 requires the proof of intention, arguably it does not dilute the strict liability principle. A reading of Article 21.2[31] along with the second paragraph of Article 2[32] establishes that strict liability is the norm. Both the articles place the responsibility of complying with the WADA Code on the athlete. The accountability of the athlete thus is absolute. This is independent of the responsibility placed on the sports federations. The sports federations have the responsibility of (1) enforcing the WADA Code and (2) educating the athletes about the WADA Code. The athlete's responsibility in that sense does not get diluted because of

23   World Anti-Doping Agency (n 16), Article 2.3
24   Ibid, Article 2.4
25   Ibid, Article 2.5
26   Ibid, Article 2.6
27   Ibid, Article 2.7
28   Ibid, Article 2.8
29   Ibid, Article 2.9
30   Ibid, Article 2.10
31   Ibid (21.2 Roles and Responsibilities of Athlete Support Personnel: 21.2.1 To be knowledgeable of and comply with all anti-doping policies and rules adopted pursuant to the Code and which are applicable to them or the athletes whom they support. . .)
32   Ibid (Article 2 Anti-Doping Rule Violations: . . . Athletes or other Persons shall be responsible for knowing what constitutes an anti-doping rule violation and the substances and methods which have been included on the Prohibited list.)

failure on the part of the sports federation to discharge their responsibilities. And that is the strict liability principle which takes into account solely the athlete's act.

In *International Olympic Committee (IOC) v. Xinyi Chen*,[33] the CAS underlined that

> Even if the Panel is willing to give the Athlete credit for being a young, honest person and her Coach credit for developing her outstanding performance results using exclusively fair and accepted training methods, such facts neither eliminate nor diminish the Athlete's duty under the IOC ADR to ensure that no Prohibited Substance enters her body, and in case of an Adverse Analytical Finding, her duty to explain the source of the Prohibited Substance.[34]

The athlete, a swimmer, tried to challenge the finding of an ADRV in this case on the basis of "substantial mistakes" committed by a WADA-accredited laboratory. However, on balance of probability the athlete was not able to prove this point.[35] The WADA Code has tried to address the criticism of strict liability by giving certain concessions to the athletes. Accordingly, the burden of proof under Article 3 of the WADA Code lays down different standards for athletes and for the federation/anti-doping organizations. Athletes are required to rebut the presumption of an ADRV or other aspects of their innocence by a balance of probability. On the other hand, the federation/anti-doping organization is required to prove an ADRV to the comfortable satisfaction of the hearing panel/tribunal. The standard of comfortable satisfaction has been stated to be greater than the balance of probability but lesser than proof beyond reasonable doubt.[36] Another concession that the WADA Code has made to soften the rigour of the strict liability principle is the incorporation of a rebuttable presumption of fault.[37] For example, in Article 3.2.2 of the

---

33 Arbitration CAS anti-doping Division (OG Rio) AD 16/005

34 Ibid para 43

35 Ibid para 47

36 World Anti-Doping Agency (n 16) (Article 3 Proof of Doping: 3.1 Burdens and Standards of Proof: The anti-doping organization shall have the burden of establishing that an anti-doping rule violation has occurred. The standard of proof shall be whether the anti-doping organization has established an anti-doping rule violation to the comfortable satisfaction of the hearing panel, bearing in mind the seriousness of the allegation which is made. This standard of proof in all cases is greater than a mere balance of probability but less than proof beyond a reasonable doubt. Where the Code places the burden of proof upon the athlete or other Person alleged to have committed an anti-doping rule violation to rebut a presumption or establish specified facts or circumstances, the standard of proof shall be by a balance of probability.). See also CAS 2010/A/2235 Union Cycliste Internationale (UCI) v. T. & Olympic Committee of Slovenia (OCS) (2011)

37 Jack Anderson, "Doping, Sport and the Law: Time for Repeal of Prohibition?" (2013) 9 (2) *International Journal of Law in Context* 135

WADA Code the presumption in favour of WADA-accredited or WADA-approved laboratories is rebuttable. Accordingly, "[t]he athlete or other [p]erson may rebut this presumption by establishing that a departure from the international Standard for Laboratories occurred which could reasonably have caused the adverse analytical finding."[38] Importantly, Article 3.1 clearly indicates that athletes can rebut the presumption of an ADRV through the balance of probability.

The other Articles of WADA Code pertaining to result management and sample analysis viz. Article 6 and Article 7, also imply rebuttable presumption of fault. In *Ihab Abdelrahman v. Egyptian NADO*,[39] the CAS noted that in order to raise a claim of an ADRV the anti-doping organization has to notify the "consequences of an AAF [Adverse Analytical Finding]."[40] Consequences of ADRVs include, amongst others, provisional suspension.[41] The mandatory requirement of notification to the athlete is in compliance with the principles of natural justice. Athletes are to be informed about the nature of ADRVs to enable them to take steps to counter the claim/rebut the presumption of doping as well as to get a provisional suspension revoked.[42] Granting of a hearing at

---

38 World Anti-Doping Agency (n 16) (3.2.2: Wada-accredited laboratories, and other laboratories approved by Wada, are presumed to have conducted Sample analysis and custodial procedures in accordance with the international Standard for Laboratories. The athlete or other Person may rebut this presumption by establishing that a departure from the international Standard for Laboratories occurred which could reasonably have caused the adverse analytical finding. If the athlete or other person rebuts the preceding presumption by showing that a departure from the international Standard for Laboratories occurred which could reasonably have caused the adverse analytical finding, then the anti-doping organization shall have the burden to establish that such departure did not cause the adverse analytical finding.)

39 CAS ad hoc Division (OG Rio) 16/023 (2016)

40 Ibid para 5.8

41 Ibid 133

42 Ibid (Article 7.3 Notification After Review Regarding Adverse Analytical Findings: if the review of an adverse analytical finding under Article 7.2 does not reveal an applicable TUE or entitlement to a TUE as provided in the International Standard for Therapeutic Use Exemptions, or departure that caused the adverse analytical finding, the anti-doping organization shall promptly notify the athlete, in the manner set out in Articles 14.1.1 and 14.1.3 and its own rules, of: (a) the adverse analytical finding; (b) the anti-doping rule violated; and (c) the athlete's right to promptly request the analysis of the B Sample or, failing such request, that the B Sample analysis may be deemed waived; (d) the scheduled date, time and place for the B Sample analysis if the athlete or anti-doping organization chooses to request an analysis of the B Sample; (e) the opportunity for the athlete and/or the athlete's representative to attend the B Sample opening and analysis within the time period specified in the international Standard for Laboratories if such analysis is requested; and (f) the athlete's right to request copies of the A and B Sample laboratory documentation package which includes information as required by the international Standard for Laboratories. if the anti-doping organization decides not to bring forward the adverse analytical finding as an anti-doping rule violation, it shall so notify the athlete and the anti-doping organizations.)

the stage of provisional suspension is also built in, which furthers the ability of the athlete to rebut the presumption of an ADVR.[43] In *Ihab Abdelrahman*,[44] the CAS notes that

> Article 7.9 of the Code sets out the Principles Applicable to Provisional Suspensions. Article 7.9.1 of the Code provides that when an AAF is received for a Prohibited Substance (that is not specified), a provisional suspension shall be imposed promptly after the review and notification. However, an athlete must be given an opportunity for a hearing on the provisional suspension.[45]

Thus in *Patrik Sinkewitz v. Union Cycliste Internationale (UCI)*,[46] Sinkewitz argued for a lifting of the provisional suspension challenging the "analyses performed on the samples he provided and the procedure which followed the reporting of the Adverse Analytical Finding."[47] Evidently the athlete denied the occurrence of the ADRV.[48] In this case, the CAS clarified that if the athlete establishes "that the apparent anti-doping rule violation has no reasonable prospects of being upheld, or that the B sample analysis does not confirm the A sample analysis"[49] provisional suspension can be lifted. Since provisional suspension is an intermediary stage, an athlete only gets an interim relief. The lifting of the provisional suspension has no bearing on the final outcome pertaining to sanctions on the non-rebuttal of an ADRV. As the CAS noted in the *Sinkewitz* case,[50] "any decision taken by this Panel with respect to the lifting of the Provisional Suspension does not affect the different question of the existence of an anti-doping rule violation (and of an alleged disciplinary responsibility of Sinkewitz) or bind any body (including any possible CAS panel at a later stage) called to adjudicate on it." Nonetheless, provision of a hearing at an intermediary stage is indicative of the modified strict liability principle that has been adopted by the WADA Code, thus incorporating flexibility.

Modified strict liability – upholding the elitist agenda?

These flexibilities do not however allow digression from the core principle of the WADA Code viz. athlete's responsibility to comply with anti-doping regulations.

43 Ibid, Article 7.9
44 Ibid
45 Ibid 7.7
46 CAS 2011/A/2479 (2011)
47 Ibid para 13
48 Ibid para 18
49 Ibid para 21
50 Ibid

This is evident from Article 9 which leads to automatic disqualification of "the result obtained in that Competition with all resulting Consequences, including forfeiture of any medals, points and prizes."[51] This is the second stage in the processes prescribed under the WADA Code. Once the ADRV is conclusively established by the anti-doping organization, there is an automatic disqualification of the individual result, in case of in-competition testing. The automatic disqualification of result and forfeiture of the medal and prize money is confined to the event in which the testing was done.[52] This rule exemplifies strict liability in its purest form. The concessions, referred to within the WADA Code, have not diluted the principle. It has softened the rigour to the extent of giving the athlete a chance to rebut the presumption of an ADRV. On the failure of the athlete to rebut the presumption of an ADRV, the result of the event gets automatically disqualified. In *A v. Fédération Internationale de Luttes Associées (FILA)*,[53] CAS justified the automatic disqualification rule by distinguishing disqualification of the results from banning an athlete. Disqualification of results essentially is about cancelling the outcome of the event in which the athlete has been proven to have used a prohibited substance or method. Banning, in contrast, is to bar participation of the athlete from all future events. Prof Kohler, Rigozzi and Prof Malinverni assert that "there is no legal or practical basis for objecting to the disqualification of an athlete who has competed with the aid of a prohibited substance, even though he or she may not have been responsible in any way whatsoever for the presence of such a substance."[54] From a non-elitist developing country perspective, this appears to be an argument of convenience.

The attempted distinction between sanction and disqualification makes no difference to an athlete in general. Disqualification of results harms the athlete's reputation and forces the athlete to challenge the ADRV findings. Evidently, as mentioned in the *Sinkewitz case*,[55] the athlete, in cases of mandatory provisional suspension, has to fight twice over: once to get the provisional suspension lifted and again to challenge the finding of an ADRV. Further, the forfeiture of prize money leads to financial loss. Finally, proving the non-existence of the ADRV itself is an arduous task. The burden placed on the athlete means that they can only challenge the cause of action viz. ADRVs under limited circumstances. First, as mentioned above, by challenging the testing procedure itself. Second, as will

51 World Anti-Doping Agency (n 16), Article 9 (An anti-doping rule violation in Individual Sports in connection with an In-Competition test automatically leads to disqualification of the result obtained in that Competition with all resulting Consequences, including forfeiture of any medals, points and prizes.)

52 Paul David, *A Guide to the World Anti-Doping Code-the Fight for the Spirit of Sport* (Cambridge University Press, 2017)

53 CAS 2001/A/317 (2001)

54 Gabrielle Kaufmann-Kohler, Antonio Rigozzi and Giorgio Malinverni, "Legal Opinion on the Conformity of Certain Provisions of the Draft World Anti-Doping Code with Commonly Accepted Principles of International Law" (2003) www.wada-ama.org/sites/default/files/resources/files/kaufmann-kohler-full.pdf (accessed 3 April 2017)

55 CAS 2011/A/2479 (n 46)

be discussed, proving therapeutic exemption and finally, though more difficult under the 2015 Code, by challenging the decision limits (to be discussed). Proving substantial errors in testing procedures requires technical expertise in addition to sound legal argument. Considering that the entire result management process is under the control of the anti-doping organization, there is an issue of conflict of interest.[56] It is the anti-doping organization which investigates, analyses and proves the ADRV through analyses of samples in laboratories accredited by WADA. The WADA Code gives the responsibility of result management to the anti-doping organization. In the whole process, with the exception of the lab which conducts the test, everything is controlled by the anti-doping organization. Understandably the anti-doping organization will seek to maximize its success rate.

Athletes are thus up against an entire system where they don't have any chance of demanding intervention by an independent body. The only option is to approach the hearing panel or the CAS after the notice of an ADRV. Hence, averting the automatic disqualification of the result by challenging the testing procedure is a daunting task for the athlete. Lack of intervention by an independent body at the stage of result management makes the task of challenging the validity of a WADA-approved test even more difficult. In *P. v. International Skating Union (ISU) & CAS 2009/A/1913 Deutsche Eisschnelllauf Gemeinschaft e.V. (DESG) v. International Skating Union (ISU)*[57] the athlete was proceeded against for an ADRV on the basis of her "blood values and profile."[58] The Athlete Biological Passport (ABP) has been developed and implemented by WADA as part of its mandate under Article 2.2. As mentioned above, Article 2.2 deals with the use or attempted use of prohibited substances or methods. The ABP enables the anti-doping organization to establish an ADRV by "indirectly reveal[ing] the effects of doping rather than attempting to detect the doping substance or method itself."[59] It involves a systematic review of the biological profile by testing the blood/urine samples of the athletes. Any significant variation in the values of the sample leads to a presumption of an ADRV under Article 2.2. Under Article 2.2 the anti-doping organization is required to prove to the comfortable satisfaction of the Panel only the use or attempted use of a prohibited substance or method. Hence, the presence of any specific substance or specific method does not need to be proven.[60] This permits more flexibility to the anti-doping organization to hold the athletes liable for anti-doping violations. Reliance on changes in biological markers, as evident from blood/urine, permits the use of circumstantial

56 Canadian Center for Ethics in Sports, "Conflict of Interest in Anti-Doping" (2016) http://cces.ca/blog/conflict-interest-anti-doping (accessed 13 April 2017)
57 CAS 2009/A/1912 (2009)
58 Ibid para 8
59 World Anti-Doping Agency, "Athlete Biological Passport" (2017) www.wada-ama.org/en/athlete-biological-passport (accessed 14 April 2017)
60 World Anti-Doping Agency, "Athlete Biological Passport Operating Guidelines" (2017) www.wada-ama.org/sites/default/files/resources/files/guidelines_abp_v6_2017_jan_en.pdf (accessed 16 April 2017)

evidence.[61] The difference being here that the circumstantial evidence relied upon is excessively technical and creates complications for athletes to rebut.

In *P. v. International Skating Union (ISU)*,[62] use of ABP as proof of an ADRV was challenged before the CAS for the first time. The concerned athlete had never tested positive on either in-competition testing or out-of-competition testing. Thus when the anti-doping organization sought to proceed against her by using ABP, she challenged the validity of ABP. However, the CAS upheld the validity of ABP as proof of an ADRV. Affirming faith in WADA as well as the scientific soundness of the test, the CAS declared that "[t]he Panel would have no hesitation in holding that new scientifically sound evidentiary methods, even not specifically mentioned in anti-doping rules, can be used at any time to investigate and discover past anti-doping rule violations that went undetected."[63] The athlete then went on to object to the processes used in the collection of the blood sample, the chain of custody, the time and place of testing, the personnel involved in collection of the blood sample and so on.[64] For example, she argued that "the phlebotomists used by the ISU at in-competition tests were not qualified for"[65] collection of blood samples. She also claimed that "the samples were not transported under proper cooling conditions and it is possible that they were affected by low temperatures."[66] The moot point of the athlete's argument was that there were deviations from the standard protocols for testing and sample collection established by the WADA Code. These protocols, being mandatory for all anti-doping organizations, were held by the CAS to not be applicable for ABP. The CAS's reasoning being that

> the WADA IST and WADA ISL, to which the ISU conforms in accordance with the ISU Anti-Doping Procedures set forth by Communication No. 1547, do not apply to blood testing done for profiling purposes, given that no complex laboratory operations are needed to analyse the blood samples and record the required hematological values.[67]

This declaration by the CAS left the athlete with a slim chance of success. Considering that an athlete was facing a career-threatening sanction did not matter to WADA or the anti-doping organization at the time.

Ironically, WADA has now integrated the entire ABP programme with the International Standard of Testing and Investigation (ISTI)[68] and the International

61 Richard H. McLaren, "Athlete Biological Passport: The Juridical Viewpoint" (2012) 4 *ISLR* 77
62 CAS 2009/A/1912 (n 57)
63 Ibid para 39
64 Ibid para 61
65 Ibid
66 Ibid para 74
67 Ibid para 65
68 World Anti-Doping Code, "International Standard for Testing and Investigation [Annex L – Results Management Requirements and Procedures for the Athlete Biological Passport]" (2017) www.wada-ama.org/sites/default/files/resources/files/2016-09-30_-_isti_final_january_2017.pdf (accessed 1 May 2017)

Standard for Laboratories (ISL).[69] Further the guidelines pertaining to operationalizing the ABP also makes it mandatory for the anti-doping organizations to follow the ISTI protocol.[70] The guidelines underline that "Only programs that fully adhere to these protocols . . . can be considered ABP Programs."[71] This change in WADA's stance might give a chance to the athlete to challenge a finding of an ADRV on the basis of ABP. It will require a lot from the athlete in terms of expertise and financial resources to counter the views of the experts who review the ABP findings. Claudia Pechstein (the athlete in the aforementioned case), could challenge her ABP due to her position. She was a five-time Olympic Gold Medalist and could afford to put up experts before the CAS who argued against the entire process used to conduct the blood profiling for ABP. Despite her efforts, she could not convince the CAS of the error in the testing process or the impact of the departures from protocols. The current ABP guidelines equally accommodate non-conformity with WADA ABP requirements viz. sample collection, transport and analysis. The guidelines permit the experts to include "all results in their review provided that their conclusions may be validly supported in the context of the non-conformity."[72] Further, the WADA Code clearly indicates that departures from protocol do not automatically lead to rejection of adverse analytical findings.[73] Coopting this point and reading it with the ABP guidelines, one can safely argue that in cases of Adverse Passport Finding (APF), departure from protocols will not lead to rejection of APF. This point is confirmed from the comment to L.1 of the ABP guidelines. The comment clarifies that

> [t]he ABP follows a similar logical structure to Results Management for analytical Testing, with both processes culminating in a possible ADRV based on, respectively, Code Article 2.2 and Code Article 2.1. An ATPF is to the ABP what an Atypical Finding (ATF) is to analytical Testing; both require further investigation. Similarly, an APF is to the ABP what the Adverse Analytical Finding (AAF) is to analytical Testing; both require Results Management in accordance with Code Article 7.

The system is not only structurally the same but procedurally also expected to follow the same protocols as provided in WADA Code Article 7. It leads to a logical conclusion that in terms of burden of proof and establishing or rebutting presumptions the parameters will be the same as for adverse analytical findings. The same is established by the CAS in *P. v. International Skating Union (ISU)*,[74] wherein it noted that the burden lies primarily on the anti-doping organization

69 World Anti-Doping Code, "International Standard for Laboratories" (2016) www.wada-ama.org/sites/default/files/resources/files/isl_june_2016.pdf (accessed 1 May 2017)

70 World Anti-Doping Agency (n 60) 25

71 Ibid

72 Ibid 114

73 Ibid (n 16)

74 CAS 2009/A/1912 (n 57)

to prove an ADRV based on ABP. Importantly, as mentioned earlier, ABP is used to prove an ADRV under Article 2.2 of the WADA Code. Hence, it follows suit that all other procedural requirements, including burden of proof, will be followed.[75] The comment to Article 2.2 permits use of ABP as one of the means through which an ADRV can be proved. This essentially legitimizes the use of ABP and puts in place the legal framework. Additionally, Article 3.2 of the WADA Code also provides that "Facts related to anti-doping rule violations may be established by any reliable means, including admissions."[76] The system thus ensures that only athletes who are up the ladder in terms of resources can fight the allegations. In *Union Cycliste Internationale (UCI) v. T. & Olympic Committee of Slovenia (OCS)*,[77] though the athlete claimed to be suffering from severe stomach problems, the UCI rejected the claim. Based on the blood profile, the expert committee unanimously decided it to be a case of "potential anti-doping rule violation."[78] Interestingly the athlete's domestic tribunal rejected the UCI's assertion and deduced the blood profile to be the result of the athlete's health condition.[79] Before the CAS, the UCI insisted that the findings of the expert committee needed to be upheld against the decision of the domestic tribunal. The UCI pointed to the CAS's lack of "scientific expertise" as the reason for giving primacy to the "appreciation of the Expert committee."[80] This line of argument reflects the problematic situation in which an athlete, and most importantly, a non-elite/developing country athlete faces. The essence of the argument being that the governing body cannot be challenged on its finding of an ADRV. Unfortunately, the CAS, too, ignored the conflict-of-*interest angle by stating that "this CAS Panel rejects the assertion, not infrequently made, both before it and (previously) before the Senate that the experts produced by UCI acted as advocates, or even accusers. UCI itself has nothing to gain from exaggerating the extent to which its sport is troubled by the scourge of doping."[81]

Accordingly, the CAS refused to question the legitimacy of the ABP as a method of proving an ADRV. For the athlete, the line of arguments based on health condition and personal circumstances clearly were no match against the

75 World Anti-Doping Agency (n 16) [Comment to Article 2.2- It has always been the case that Use or Attempted Use of a Prohibited Substance or Prohibited Method may be established by any reliable means. As noted in the Comment to Article 3.2, unlike the proof required to establish an anti-doping rule violation under Article 2.1, Use or Attempted Use may also be established by other reliable means such as admissions by the Athlete, witness statements, documentary evidence, conclusions drawn from longitudinal profiling, including data collected as part of the Athlete Biological Passport, or other analytical information which does not otherwise satisfy all the requirements to establish "Presence" of a Prohibited Substance under Article 2.1.]

76 Ibid, Article 3.2

77 CAS 2010/A/2235 (2011)

78 Ibid 7

79 Ibid 8

80 Ibid, para 27

81 Ibid para 29

expert committee. The CAS was not convinced that chronic gastric problems or prolonged exposure to "altitude training" or treatment for wasp biting or the birth of his second child and related distress, was the reason for the fluctuating blood profile. Clearly in the absence of strong rebuttal through independent scientific evidence, the arguments are inane. The burden of proof thus can hardly ever be discharged unless one can come up with a team of world-class scientists and expert evidence. And that, in the absence of *pro bono* litigation, is all about deep pockets and abundant resources. For an elite athlete, having access to both gives a better fighting chance. In the absence of the same, which will be the case in the majority of disputes, the consequences are severe, as noted above. In the case of ABP findings, another problematic aspect is the inherent contradiction in the philosophy that justifies automatic disqualification. As discussed, automatic disqualification of the result is justified on the basis of unfair competitive advantage to the delinquent athlete vis-á-vis others. The level playing field is an argument used to support the automatic disqualification of results.[82] However, as noted by the CAS in *Union Cycliste Internationale (UCI) v. T. & Olympic Committee of Slovenia (OCS)*[83] in cases of ABP the automatic disqualification of results is more difficult to justify as "it is not easy in a case such as the present to identify in connection with which events the Athlete's doping violation occurred."[84] This is because unlike the analytical findings based on the presence of a specific substance/method, ABP findings are about process based on "individual, electronic record for each athlete, in which the results of all doping tests over a period of time are collated."[85] Evidently then, all ABP does is widen the net to catch all athletes for all possible breaches.[86] In the absence of resources enabling the athletes to rebut the findings of the profiling, the ADRV is a foregone conclusion. As will be seen subsequently, the defenses against sanction (and not disqualification) are equally problematic in terms of evidence and proof. The cases where the athletes have been successful in challenging the tests are far and few between.

Testing the tests: impossible dream for the non-elites?

Modahl v. British Athletic Federation Limited[87] is a classic pre-WADA case which gives insight into the difficulties of challenging the tests or the processes. Though the case was about alleged breach of contract by the British Athletic Federation

82 Gabrielle Kaufmann-Kohler, Antonio Rigozzi and Giorgio Malinverni (n 54)
83 Ibid
84 Ibid para 65
85 Ibid 3
86 Matthew Hard, "Caught in the Net: Athletes' Rights and the World Anti-Doping Agency" (2010) 19 *Southern California Interdisciplinary Law Journal* 533
87 [1999] UKHL 37 www.publications.parliament.uk/pa/ld199899/ldjudgmt/jd990722/modahl.htm (accessed 15 May 2017)

(BAF), its genesis rested in the disputed lab test. Modhal was suspended by BAF for having committed an ADRV. On a subsequent appeal, she was acquitted of the charges of doping. The independent tribunal raised doubt about the veracity of the lab tests. On being reinstated, Modhal sued the BAF for compensation due to breach of contract. She claimed "that her suspension and the initiation of disciplinary proceedings were in breach of the contract between her and the BAF. . . . She claims damages for the financial loss she suffered because for nearly a year she was unable to compete in international athletics."[88] The argument was that the BAF suspended Modhal by relying on a test conducted by a non-accredited laboratory. Modhal argued that the lab, which was accredited by the IOC, lost its accreditation when "it had moved its premises without notifying the IOC or IAAF."[89] This was understandably an argument of desperation. As the House of Lords states, there cannot logically be any effect on accreditation of a lab by shifting of premises. Lord Hoffmann remarked,

> I must confess that I would find it remarkable if it did [the shifting of the premises leading to revocation of accreditation]. The IOC has procedures for the regular checking of accredited laboratories and a removal to less suitable premises could well be a ground for the IOC revoking an accreditation. The same might be true of changes in personnel or equipment. But I find it hard to see why such matters should ipso facto nullify the accreditation without any act on the part of the IOC.[90]

Lord Hoffman further observed that "the fact that the laboratory was not accredited does not necessarily mean that the test was wrong."[91] Essentially accreditation or lack of it was regarded as inconsequential in the outcome of the test result. The other angle was complete lack of accountability that was expected from the National Federation. Lord Hoffman insisted that the concerned lab was under the jurisdiction of the Portugal Athletic Federation (PAF), and hence the BAF could not be expected to have knowledge of the accreditation status. Since Modhal was tested during her participation in an athletic competition in Lisbon, PAF was responsible for conducting the tests.

As per Lord Hoffman, the BAF's role was confined to act on the finding of a positive result in a foreign country. The BAF was required by the IAAF to suspend the athlete and initiate disciplinary proceedings. Accordingly, non-accreditation of the lab which tested the sample is not a matter of concern for a National Federation like BAF. This approach of the House of Lords raises questions as to the futility of accreditation. It also raises questions about the safeguards available to protect the interest of athletes. The current anti-doping regime under

88 Ibid
89 Ibid
90 Ibid
91 Ibid

the WADA Code makes it clear that WADA-accredited or WADA-approved labs are presumed to have followed the established protocols for conducting tests. Rebuttal of this presumption can be given if it is proven that deviation from protocols led to the positive finding. In such a case, the anti-doping organization/ federation can counter by proving that deviations did not affect the test and then the test result is validated.[92] Article 6 of the WADA Code makes testing by an accredited or approved laboratory mandatory only for Article 2.1 violations viz. presence of prohibited substance or method.[93] Thus to prove use or attempted use of prohibited substance or method, for example, "analytical results" from a non-accredited or non-approved lab can be used. This approach can be justified on the basis that, apart from Article 2.1 violations, other violations can be proved on the basis of non-analytical findings, and analytical results are only used to strengthen the case. Thus, on paper, athletes currently have a better system than Modhal, because tests by an accredited/approved laboratory are a must. However, as the Russian doping scandal revealed, accreditation itself is not a guarantee against manipulation of samples. Athletes continue to face the problem that Modhal faced – how to disprove the tests? The discussion so far has revealed the nearly impossible task of countering the analytical as well as the non-analytical findings. The WADA Code also permits acceptance of analytical results notwithstanding deviation from established protocols. This means that a laboratory can be accredited or approved, but has the flexibility of deviating from the International Standards.

The cost of proving the tests wrong is immense, even if judged from a balance of probability standard. Modhal, for example, had to sell her house to fight the case against the BAF.[94] With the CAS in place, athletes from the First World might find it less costly, but for the developing country/non-elite athletes defending before the CAS is financially onerous. Apart from travel costs and costs for a lawyer, there are additional costs for experts and other evidence. Though the CAS has provisions for legal aid,[95] the challenge of testing the test remains a fundamental problem. Since developing country/non-elite athletes have to overcome circumstances based on socio-economic concerns, thinking of a nuanced approach to rebut the findings of an ADRV remains a challenge. Hence, legal aid

92 World Anti-Doping Agency (n 16), Article 3.2.2
93 Ibid, Article 6 (6.1 Use of Accredited and Approved Laboratories: For purposes of Article 2.1, Samples shall be analysed only in Wada-accredited laboratories or laboratories otherwise approved by Wada. The choice of the WADA-accredited or Wada-approved laboratory used for the Sample analysis shall be determined exclusively by the anti-doping organization responsible for results management.)
94 Edward Procter, "Dispute Resolution in Sport: The Role of Sport Resolutions (United Kingdom)" (2010) 1 *Comment ISLR* www.sportresolutions.co.uk/uploads/related-documents/Dispute_Resolution_in_Sport_-_The_Role_of_Sport_Resolutions_UK.pdf (accessed 17 May 2017)
95 International Council of Arbitration for Sport, "Guidelines on Legal Aid Before the Court of Arbitration for Sport" (2016) www.tas-cas.org/fileadmin/user_upload/Legal_Aid_Rules_2016_English.pdf (accessed 17 May 2017)

at the stage of litigation is welcome, but one is arguing for more accountability at the beginning of the anti-doping process. Hence, condonation of deviations by accredited/approved labs, within the WADA Code is a problem. It raises barriers to accessing a fair and equitable chance of rebuttal. The system thus creates complications for the non-elites/developing country athletes. It also equips athletes with better access to resources to take on the system. The Lance Armstrong case is a classic example as to what an elite, resource-rich athlete can do to con the system. As per the US Anti-Doping Agency (USADA) "[Lance Armstrong case is an example of] a massive team doping scheme, more extensive than any revealed in professional sports history."[96] Hence, a closer look at the method of challenging the correctness of the lab tests is important. *Vadim Devyatovskiy v. IOC et al.*[97] is a rare example where the athletes were able to successfully challenge the tests. Vadim Devyatovskiy and Ivan Tsikhan were two Belarusian hammer throwers who tested positive for testosterone. The tests were conducted by the Beijing lab as part of the anti-doping measures carried out during the 2008 Beijing Olympics. The athletes challenged the "validity of the analyses conducted by the Beijing Laboratory."[98] The points on which they challenged the tests are reflective of the nuanced approach needed in such cases.

The IOC DC rejected the challenge and found the athletes guilty of having committed an ADRV. In their appeal, the athletes pointed out that:

1   Since the B sample analysis was carried out by the same "Laboratory analyst who was also 'heavily involved' in the analysis of each Athlete's A Sample who conducted A sample analysis,"[99] it violated the WADA-mandated ISL.
2   The B sample test, thus being void, did not confirm the A sample test, and hence the positive finding stands cancelled.
3   There was a failure of quality-control checks during A and B sample analysis.
4   A defective mass spectrometry test was conducted in violation of ISL.
5   Incomplete information was given in the documentation pertaining to the lab tests.
6   There was clear evidence of human error and defective equipment.

On the whole, the athletes contended that "the IOC has failed to discharge its burden of proof" *because the results* "are simply insufficiently reliable to lead the Panel to have comfortable satisfaction that an anti-doping rule violation has occurred."[100] Importantly, they insisted that the ISL is a fundamental safeguard of the athlete's rights. This mirrors the argument of Modhal, who insisted that tests

---

96   Reasoned Decision of the United States Anti-Doping Agency on Disqualification and Ineligibility, United States Anti-Doping Agency, Claimant v. Lance Armstrong, Respondent (2012) https://d3epuodzu3wuis.cloudfront.net/ReasonedDecision.pdf
97   CAS 2009/A/1752 Vadim Devyatovskiy v/ IOC; CAS 2009/A/1753 Ivan Tsikhan v/ IOC
98   Ibid para 2.9
99   Ibid para 3.12
100 Ibid para 3.120

by an accredited lab were fundamental to safeguarding the rights of the athlete.[101] They also challenged the legitimacy of the burden placed on the athlete to rebut the presumption under Article 3.2.2. As stated above the athlete is required to prove "by a balance of probability, a departure from the International Standard for Laboratories that could reasonably have caused the Adverse Analytical Finding."[102] Creating a reasonable doubt about the test is indeed a problematic requirement, and hence the athletes argued that one should only prove departure from ISL.

Indeed, under the 2003 WADA Code, the athlete could rebut the presumption in favour of the tests by "establishing that a departure from the International Standard occurred."[103] The subsequent revisions, including the 2015 version, expanded the burden of proof of the athlete. Since the 2008 Beijing Olympics were governed by the 2003 Code, the athletes insisted that their burden of proof could not be reversed/expanded. The athletes also raised the conflict of interest aspect by pointing out that

> the IOC Executive Board was in charge of the anti-doping policy at the Games. The IOC, they aver, is the entity bearing ultimate responsibility for the anti-doping program. From the point of view of the Appellants, both the BOCOG (Beijing Organizing Committee for the Games) and the Beijing laboratory are agents of the IOC with respect to the anti-doping policy.[104]

Clearly the athletes were urging the CAS to reject the test results on the aforementioned grounds. The IOC expectedly kept on harping on ISL compliance and validity of the test results.

The CAS first had to resolve the conflict between the 2003 WADA Code and the 2008 IOC anti-doping rules (IOC ADR 2008), which were applied to the Beijing games and the case. The IOC ADR 2008 had been amended to incorporate the expanded burden of proof on the athletes. Thus, the IOC ADR 2008 required the athlete to rebut the presumption in favour of tests by raising reasonable doubt about the outcome. This clearly was in contradiction to the 2003 version of the WADA Code. Because the IOC was mandated to comply with the WADA Code applicable during the Beijing Olympics, the validity of the IOC ADR 2008 was doubtful. Further, the IOC ADR 2008 itself had contradictory provisions wherein it made the Code as well as the ADR mandatory. However, in terms of primacy and hierarchy of authorities, the IOC itself insisted that the WADA Code was supreme. For the CAS the resolution of the conflict had to be in favour of the athletes by insisting that the WADA Code 2003 would override the IOC ADR 2008. The legal principle the CAS referred to in support of this conclusion was "that an accused party can be tried and

101 [1999] UKHL 3 (n 87)

102 World Anti-Doping Agency (n 16), Comment to Article 3.2.2

103 World Anti-Doping Agency-Play True, "World Anti-Doping Code" (2003) www.wada-ama.org/sites/default/files/resources/files/wada_code_2003_en.pdf (accessed 13 May 2017)

104 CAS 2009/A/1752 (n 97)

sanctioned only under the laws which governed at the time the offending act was committed, the exception being the principle of lex mitior, is a fundamental principle of law which is accepted by the majority of national jurisdictions, including Switzerland."[105] The CAS also referred to the principle of "contra proferentem, i.e., to the detriment of the promulgator of the conflicting or contradictory provision."[106] The next issue that the CAS had to deal with was that of disputed tests and their outcome. Understandably the burden under the 2003 WADA Code was easier for an athlete to discharge as it required only proof of deviation from the ISL. This was also in consonance with the "purpose, scope and organization of the world anti-doping program and the code,"[107] wherein it is emphatically stated that "[a]dherence to the International Standards is mandatory for compliance with the Code."[108] Accordingly, the only thing the CAS had to judge was whether the athletes had "succeeded in establishing on the 'balance of probability' that the Beijing Laboratory departed from the ISLs in its performance of the IRMS analysis."[109] Analysing the manner in which the Beijing lab conducted the isotope-ratio mass spectrometry (IRMS) test, the CAS concluded that "on the balance of probability, several of the values measured in each of the Athlete's IRMS analysis do indeed fall outside of the Laboratory's acceptable range, whatever that range may be."[110] The CAS was equally critical of the manner in which the samples were handled and placed in the "auto sampler" noting that "the interruption of the preprogrammed sequence for testing in order to (manually) alter the positioning of the vials in their respective slots poses the risk that the results obtained for one sample will be incorrectly attributed to another sample."[111] Further, the CAS raised concerns with regards to the quality of the test by holding that "the Panel is troubled by the incomplete explanation of why the Laboratory chose to alter the Sequence File for inclusion in the Documentation Packages."[112] Accordingly, the CAS was convinced and agreed with the athletes that "the failure of the Laboratory to properly record the 'mid-stream' interruption and changes made in the sequencing of the vials for IRMS analysis constituted a 'departure' from the ISL."[113]

On the issue of quality control the CAS also held that "the Beijing Laboratory did not, at the time of the analysis, properly document the quality control procedures, in particular, the failure of the positive control and the use of the

105 Ibid para 4.27
106 Ibid para 4.28
107 World Anti-Doping Agency (n 16)
108 Ibid 12
109 CAS 2009/A/1752 (n 97) para 5.52
110 Ibid para 5.59
111 Ibid para 5.104
112 Ibid para 5.111
113 Ibid para 5.124

internal standards, in accordance with ISL."[114] Though this was not regarded as significant, because flexibilities exist to ensure quality control in various other ways, the CAS strongly disapproved of the use of the same person to analyse the A and B samples and held that

> analyst involved in the "A" sample analysis, regardless of whether the activity of that analyst does or does not involve direct interaction with the open or accessible sample or aliquot, may not be involved in any activity with regard to the "B" sample analysis which involves direct interaction with the open or accessible "B" sample or aliquot.[115]

Having gone through all the arguments and counterarguments, the CAS concluded that:

1   With respect to Devyatovskij, the "[r]espondent (IOC) could not prove to the comfortable satisfaction of the Panel that the variability in his 'B' sample IRMS results were reliable."[116]
2   With respect to Tsikhan, the CAS "was persuaded to its comfortable satisfaction that the analytical results confirmed the exogenous source of the testosterone . . . [H]owever, the mere fact of an Adverse Analytical Finding does not permit the Respondent (IOC) to rely solely on the Laboratory's positive analysis to discharge its burden of proof."[117]
3   Conclusive proof of "violations of the Laboratory's documentation and reporting requirements of ISL . . . in addition to a violation of the 'Different Analysts' rule."[118]
4   Infringement of "transparency and verification of the testing process"[119] that "represent fundamental rights of the athlete."[120]
5   Violation of the different analyst rule (as was required under the ISL 2003) was regarded as a breach of safeguards provided to the athletes.

The CAS decided the matter in favour of the athletes by nullifying the tests reiterating that

> Doping is an offence which requires the application of strict rules. If an athlete is to be sanctioned solely on the basis of the provable presence of a prohibited substance in his body, it is his or her fundamental right to know that

114 Ibid para 5.137
115 Ibid para 5.173
116 Ibid para 6.2
117 Ibid para 6.3
118 Ibid para 6.4
119 Ibid para 6.7
120 Ibid

the Respondent, as the Testing Authority, including the WADA-accredited laboratory working with it, has strictly observed the mandatory safeguards.[121]

Clearly this is a different take from the current anti-doping regime, which has upped the ante for the athletes. As the above details show, the athletes could win the case purely on the lower burden of proof viz. to show only deviation from ISL. Further, the ISL 2003 made it clear that A and B samples could not be analysed by the same person. ISL 2016, for example, has no rule pertaining to different analysts. These differences enabled the athletes to argue the case better. Under the 2015 WADA Code, the athlete has to prove a lot more to question the tests; hence, as already stated, there is a remote chance of success on this ground. From a non-elite/developing country perspective this renders the presumption in favour of the tests as good as irrefutable, and effectively cancels out the flexibilities of a modified strict liability regime.

The curious case of therapeutic use exemption: an elite luxury

The other grounds on which the athlete can avoid the blame of an ADRV is the therapeutic use exemption (TUE). This exemption permits the athlete to use prohibited substances/methods under strict conditions. The underlying consideration for the grant of TUEs is the treatment of an athlete's medical condition without enhancing performance. The International Standard for Therapeutic Use Exemption (ISTUE) prescribes the criterion to be strictly followed in assessing a TUE application. Thus, an athlete has to show, by balance of probability, that

a. The Prohibited Substance or Prohibited Method in question is needed to treat an acute or chronic medical condition, such that the Athlete would experience a significant impairment to health if the Prohibited Substance or Prohibited Method were to be withheld. b. The Therapeutic Use of the Prohibited Substance or Prohibited Method is highly unlikely to produce any additional enhancement of performance beyond what might be anticipated by a return to the Athlete's normal state of health following the treatment of the acute or chronic medical condition. c. There is no reasonable Therapeutic alternative to the Use of the Prohibited Substance or Prohibited Method. d. The necessity for the Use of the Prohibited Substance or Prohibited Method is not a consequence, wholly or in part, of the prior Use (without a TUE) of a substance or method which was prohibited at the time of such Use.[122]

121 Ibid para 6.10
122 World Anti-Doping Code, "International Standard-Therapeutic Use Exemptions" (2016), Article 4.1 www.wada-ama.org/sites/default/files/resources/files/wada-2016-istue-final-en_0.pdf (accessed 12 May 2017)

Therefore, the proof of the athlete's medical condition is *sine qua non* for applying for a TUE. Additionally, the lack of alternative treatment is also an important aspect of the TUE application process. It is important to note that athletes need to prove their inability to participate in competitive sport without the TUE. In other words, the medical ailment is presumed to have diminished their ability to compete. They can also prove that competing with the ailment is life-threatening. The exemption is sought then to enable the affected athlete to compete by enhancing the performance to normal levels.

This justification for TUE is problematic in view of the principled objection to the use of performance-enhancing drugs/methods. Permitting TUEs to enhance performance to normal level leads to a debate on identifying the normal level itself. The debate in Dutee Chand[123] brings forth starkly the problem of defining what normal/natural is. Challenging the legality of the IAAF-mandated Hyperandrogenism Regulations, Dutee argued that high testosterone levels in some female athletes due to genetic traits was normal. This genetic trait was inborn and comparable to other inborn and unusual traits like height, lung capacity, foot size or visual acuity that some athletes have.[124] For example, LeBron James is regarded as one of the greatest basketball players because "[h]is body (6-foot-8, 250 pounds) allows him to dunk a basketball 3 ½ feet away from the rim. His legs give him the capability to produce 700 pounds of pressure per leap."[125] Further, she pointed out that "no testosterone limit [is] applicable to male athletes. Male athletes with testosterone level falling above the upper limit of the 'normal' range of male testosterone are permitted to compete."[126] In the context of TUE, therefore, proving the normal competency level is a subjective task. The ISTUE does not define the word "normal." If an athlete is suffering from an ailment, it is impossible to fathom the athlete's normal state. Further, comparing with other "normal" athletes is problematic in view of the fact that some may have unusual genetic traits. Mulhall puts forth the problematic aspect of the word "normal" thus:

> an athlete who suffers a reduction of natural testosterone due to testicular cancer would be allowed to use that substance from an external source to return to a state of "normal" health. Does "normal" mean normal for that athlete or within the range of normal for males of the human race? It may be that there is no reliable record of "normal" for a particular athlete prior to the athlete's illness. Further, "normal" hormonal levels in each individual vary over time. So the only available criterion may be the range of "normal"

123 CAS 2014/A/3759 Dutee Chand v Athletics Federation of India (AFI) & The International Association of Athletics Federations (IAAF)
124 Ibid para 113
125 Karl Ekwurtzel, "Why You're Not an Olympian: Athletes Built for Their Sports" *ABC News* (New York, 7 August 2012) http://abcnews.go.com/Sports/olympics/olympic-physiques-michael-phelps-usain-bolt-athletes-built/story?id=16917476 (accessed 15 May 2017)
126 CAS 2014/A/3759 (n 123) para 114

for all (male) humans who have been tested. In that circumstance the athlete would only have to ensure his enhanced testosterone levels are within the "normal" range, and he could be near or at the top of that range without violating the Code. On the other hand, an athlete who has not suffered from a testosterone-reducing disease is not permitted to increase "low-normal" levels of his testosterone to at or near the top of the normal range.[127]

From a non-elite/developing country perspective, the word "normal" thus stratifies physiological hierarchies. Since, as noted by Mulhall, there is ambiguity in the process of determining what is normal, a non-elite/developing country athlete will be caught in the web of confusing information in proving their normal state.

The problem of accessibility to resources also diminishes the chances of a non-elite athlete ever matching the efforts of an elite athlete for getting a TUE. Kayser, Mauron and Miah argue that "depending on their nationality and sports speciality, athletes may differ enormously with regard to their access to care, supervision, and a high quality medical and technological environment."[128] Article 6.6 of the ISTUE clearly states that "Any costs incurred by the Athlete in making the TUE application and in supplementing it as required by the TUEC are the responsibility of the Athlete."[129] The stakes are therefore quite high for a non-elite/developing country athlete. The non-elite/developing country athlete, in addition, will have to bear the cost of proving a comparable parameter for establishing their normal state. Apart from the theoretical and resource impediments listed above, there is another more problematic aspect of the TUE. From 13 September 2016 to 3 October 2016 a group of hackers called Fancy Bear leaked several athletes' confidential data.[130] They hacked the WADA database and leaked athletes' TUE data, among other information.[131] The data pertained to high-profile athletes like Olympic Gold Medalist Simone Biles, tennis superstar Serena Williams and others.[132] The allegations were that TUEs were being abused by those who could, and that is the current theme of discussion within the sporting world viz. the abuse of the TUE. The use of TUEs by high-performing athletes like Williams and Biles might on the face appear proper and in accordance with the rule. However,

127 Stephen J. Mulhall, "A Critique of the World Anti-Doping Code" (2006) 64 *Advocate Vancouver* 29

128 Bengt Kayser, Alexander Mauron and Andy Miah, "Current Anti-Doping Policy: A Critical Appraisal" BMC *Medical Ethics* (2007) https://bmcmedethics.biomedcentral.com/articles/10.1186/1472-6939-8-2 (accessed 19 May 2015)

129 World Anti-Doping Code (n 122) 14

130 World Anti-Doping Agency-play True, "Frequently Asked Questions (FAQ)-Therapeutic Use Exemptions (TUEs)" (17 November 2011) www.wada-ama.org/sites/default/files/resources/files/2016-11-17-qa_tues_en.pdf (accessed 19 May 2017)

131 Fancy Bears' Hack Team, "American Athletes Caught Doping 2016–09–13" https://fancybear.net/pages/1.html (accessed 15 May 2017)

132 Gillian Mohney, "Simone Biles' ADHD Meds Among Common Drugs Banned from Olympics" *ABC News* (New York, 14 September 2016) http://abcnews.go.com/Health/simone-biles-adhd-meds-common-drugs-banned-olympics/story?id=42081189 (accessed 18 May 2017)

the concern relates to the fairness of the TUE process in view of the fact that most of the athletes dominating the sporting world are coincidentally also the beneficiary of a TUE. The list, as revealed from the hack, includes Olympians (data pertained to 2016 Rio Olympics) all of whom, barring a few, are from the developed countries.[133] This raises questions about the integrity of the TUE process as well as the ease with which the elites are granted TUEs. If a large number of Olympians are using TUEs and giving winning performances, it forces one to question the role of WADA as well as the role of anti-doping organizations.[134] The TUE application process is initiated by the athlete and vetted by the concerned National/International Federation.[135] WADA's role is only to review the decisions to grant or not to grant the TUE, as and when the matter is referred to it.[136] Thus, the TUE process is decentralized, with WADA having a limited role.

WADA does however have a right to *suo moto* review a TUE decision, and that is an important aspect.[137] This allows WADA to monitor the TUEs granted and intervene to stop their abuse. The latest controversy on TUEs has put WADA on the defensive. WADA has admitted to a phenomenal increase in TUEs between 2014 and 2016 viz. 48 percent. WADA justifies this increase as a "direct result of an increase of TUEs being entered into ADAMS and not an increase in TUE applications."[138] The Anti-Doping Administration & Management System (ADAMS) is "[w]eb-based database management tool for data entry, storage, sharing, and reporting designed to assist stakeholders and WADA in their anti-doping operations."[139] WADA has made it mandatory for all anti-doping organizations to record TUE information with ADAMS since 2016. WADA cited this as one of the contributing factors for the 48 percent increase in TUEs. This automatically leads to the question of how monitoring was being performed prior to 2016. Does it mean that WADA was not rigorous enough in monitoring the TUE processes? With a large number of high-profile dominant athletes/sportspersons enjoying TUEs, does it indicate that pre-2016 TUEs were

---

133 Andy Brown, "Fancy Bears Hack: 107 Athletes; 23 Countries; 25 Sports" (2016) www.sportsintegrityinitiative.com/fancy-bears-hack-107-athletes-23-countries-25-sports/ (accessed 20 May 2017); See also Jeff Powell, "WADA Appear to Keep Doling Out Therapeutic Use Exemptions Like Sweeties to Children . . . 53 of Our Olympians Were Using Them (and that's just the Brits!)" *Mail Online* (London, 16 September 2016) www.dailymail.co.uk/sport/other-sports/article-3792069/WADA-appear-doling-Therapeutic-Use-Exemptions-like-sweeties-children-53-Olympians-using-s-just-Brits.html (accessed 21 May 2017)

134 Sean Ingle, "Wada Hacking Scandal: Debate Turns to the Use of Powerful Legal Drugs-condemnation of Hackers Is Followed by Questions Regarding the Processes of Applying for and Taking Certain Therapeutic Remedies" *The Guardian* (London, 15 September 2016) www.theguardian.com/sport/2016/sep/14/wada-hacking-abuse-debate-theraputic-use-drugs (accessed 21 May 2017)

135 World Anti-Doping Agency (n 16) Article 4.4.2–4.4.3

136 Ibid, Article 4.4.3.2 and 4.4.6

137 Ibid, Article 4.4.6–4.4.7

138 World Anti-Doping Agency-play True (n 130) para 15

139 World Anti-Doping Code (n 122) 5

being abused?[140] As of now the answers to these questions are not forthcoming from WADA, but there are allegations of TUE abuse. Since the decision to grant TUEs rests with the national/international sports governing bodies there is always a likelihood of bias. Especially in the context of elite athletes, the sport's governing bodies are likely to be lax in strictly implementing the ISTUE guidelines. The clearest evidence of such a bias is found in the report of the Cycling Independent Reform Commission (CIRC).[141] The CIRC was constituted by UCI to "investigate whether UCI officials directly contributed to the development of a culture of doping in cycling, in particular by mismanaging the testing and/or by covering up positive tests, and whether the UCI and other governing bodies and officials were implicated in ineffective investigation of doping practices."[142] In the course of its investigation the CIRC reported on the abuse of TUEs. For the purpose of present discussion this is the part that will be focused upon. With regards to TUEs, the CIRC recorded statements of riders admitting the ease with which TUEs are obtained for banned substances like steroids. The CIRC found evidence that the TUE programme was being systematically abused to enhance performance. As the CIRC noted "90% of TUEs were used for performance-enhancing purposes."[143] The CIRC also found that the TUE Committee (TUEC), constituted by the UCI, was defunct. Instead, all the TUE decisions were being made by individual doctors of UCI.[144]

This finding was based on the report prepared by the Institute of National Anti-Doping Organizations (iNADO).[145] This practice was a clear procedural infringement of ISTUE Article 5.2. The article makes it mandatory for all National/International Sports Federations to have a TUEC.[146] Further, Article 5.3 of the ISTUE states that

> Each National Anti-Doping Organization, International Federation and Major Event Organization must establish a clear process for applying to its TUEC for a TUE that complies with the requirements of this International Standard. It must also publish details of that process by (at a minimum) posting the information in a conspicuous place on its website and sending the information to WADA. WADA may re-publish the same information on its own website.[147]

140 Andy Brown (n 133)
141 Dr Dick Marty, Mr Peter Nicholson, Prof Dr Ulrich Haas, "Cycling Independent Reform Commission-Report to the President of the Union Cycliste Internationale" (2015) www.uci.ch/mm/Document/News/CleanSport/16/87/99/CIRCReport2015_Neutral.pdf (accessed 22 May 2017)
142 Ibid 16
143 Ibid 61
144 Ibid 154
145 For more information on iNADO see www.inado.org/home.html (accessed 23 May 2017)
146 World Anti-Doping Code (n 122) Article 5.2 12 [Each National Anti-Doping Organization, International Federation and Major Event Organization must establish a TUEC to consider whether applications for grant or recognition of TUEs meet the conditions set out in Article 4.1]
147 Ibid 12

By rendering the UCI TUEC defunct, there was no possibility of complying with the requirement of Article 5.3 of the ISTUE or with the requirement of Article 5.4.[148] This reaffirms the conflict-of-interest argument noted above. The larger issue though is the inaction on the part of WADA in reviewing the TUE. As has been noted, WADA has a supervisory role in the TUE process and does not itself grant TUEs. It is required to review TUE decisions either *suo moto* or on applications for the same by the athletes or the governing bodies/anti-doping organization.[149] The CIRC report points out WADA's failure in performing this crucial role. The TUE granted to Chris Froome in 2014 by UCI is cited by the CIRC report as an example of such laxities. Chris Froome, the three-time Tour de France winner, was granted a TUE issued not by a "TUE Committee, but by a single UCI staff member."[150] Though the TUE was properly reported in the ADAMS, WADA forwent the chance of reviewing the TUE process and reversing UCI's decision. Interestingly, Chris Froome is one of the athletes whose TUE record was leaked by Fancy Bear.[151] From a non-elite/developing country perspective the issue is not whether the elite athletes have abused TUE, it is the larger issue of the potentiality of abuse taking place in practice through systemic failures, as highlighted in the CIRC report. Logic and experience both indicate that the relaxations will be in favour of those who are elite and are dominant sport personalities. In the case of the UCI, the CIRC report documents the various relaxations in rules that were made to accommodate Lance Armstrong. The CIRC document clearly puts the onus on UCI for allowing Armstrong to get away with doping.[152]

A Serena Williams or Simone Biles or any other high-profile elite athlete, having the best available resources, is bound to be aided by their federation through a

---

148 Ibid, Article 5.4 [Each National Anti-Doping Organization, International Federation and Major Event Organization must promptly report (in English or French) all decisions of its TUEC granting or denying TUEs, and all decisions to recognize or refusing to recognize other Anti-Doping Organizations' TUE decisions, through ADAMS or any other system approved by WADA. In respect of TUEs granted, the information reported shall include (in English or French): 13 2016 ISTUE – 20 November 2015 a. not only the approved substance or method, but also the dosage(s), frequency and route of Administration permitted, the duration of the TUE, and any conditions imposed in connection with the TUE; and b. the TUE application form and the relevant clinical information (translated into English or French) establishing that the Article 4.1 conditions have been satisfied in respect of such TUE (for access only by WADA, the Athlete's National Anti-Doping Organization and International Federation, and the Major Event Organization organizing an Event in which the Athlete wishes to compete).]

149 Ibid, Article 8.0

150 Dr Dick Marty, Mr Peter Nicholson, Prof Dr Ulrich Haas (n 144) 154

151 Guardian Sport, "Froome and Wiggins Defend TUEs Use as Team GB Athletes Warned Over Leaks" (London, 15 September 2016) www.theguardian.com/sport/2016/sep/15/chris-froome-defends-use-tues-wada-hacking-leaks (accessed 25 May 2017)

152 Dr Dick Marty, Mr Peter Nicholson, Prof Dr Ulrich Haas (n 144) 173

less stringent application of ISTUE.[153] Additionally, one will have to depend on WADA to be vigilant enough to review closely the TUE process. In the absence of any specific application for review, the only hope is a *suo moto* review by WADA. And there is no binding obligation on WADA to go for a *suo moto* review under the WADA Code.[154] Hence the provision of TUE itself becomes a problematic aspect and contributes to engendering and propagating the elitist agenda within sport. That TUEs are difficult to monitor and susceptible to abuse was argued for a long time by the IOC. Reinold points out that the "most important reason for the lack of rules [pertaining to medical exemption or therapeutic use] seemed to be the Commission's [IOC Medical Commission] fear that medical use exemptions would open up loopholes for cheaters using substances not for therapy, as claimed, but for performance enhancement."[155] Sports scientist Ross Tucker has gone on record to argue that all TUEs should be banned "in competition."[156] Ironically, a review of the TUE disputes decided by CAS gives the indication of a situation where the governing bodies/anti-doping agencies can make the granting of a TUE extremely difficult. As argued above, such stringency will be largely applied to non-elites/developing country athletes for two reasons. First, non-elite/developing country athletes lack the resources to convince the TUEC of the genuineness of the TUE application. Second, there are hardly any compelling reasons for the governing bodies/anti-doping organizations to be flexible on the rules for these same athletes. The cases reviewed hereafter will reveal that once the TUEC decides, the chances of winning before the CAS and getting a favourable decision are almost non-existent for the athlete. In *WADA v. USADA & Scherf*,[157] there was confusion galore about the TUE status. The key points, in the context of the present discussion, pertain to the athlete's background, the role of the national anti-doping organization and the communication gap between the

153 Mens Tennis Forum, "2015 CIRC Report: Therapeutic Use Exemptions (TUEs) Are Abused" (2016) www.menstennisforums.com/2-general-messages/835241-2015-circ-report-therapeutic-use-exemptions-tues-abused.html (accessed 27 May 2017)

154 World Anti-Doping Agency (n 16), [Article 4.4.6: Article WADA must review an International Federation's decision not to recognize a TUE granted by the National Anti-Doping Organization that is referred to it by the athlete or the athlete's National Anti-Doping Organization. in addition, WADA must review an International Federation's decision to grant a TUE that is referred to it by the athlete's National Anti-Doping Organization. WADA may review any other TUE decisions at any time, whether upon request by those affected or on its own initiative. If the TUE decision being reviewed meets the criteria set out in the International Standard for Therapeutic Use Exemptions, WADA will not interfere with it. If the TUE decision does not meet those criteria, WADA will reverse it.]

155 Marcel Reinold, "Arguing Against Doping: A Discourse Analytical Study on Olympic Anti-Doping Between the 1960s and the Late 1980s" (2012) *International Olympic Committee Postgraduate Research Grant Programme 2011 Final Research Report* https://library.olympic.org/Default/doc/SYRACUSE/62313/arguing-against-doping-a-discourse-analytical-study-on-olympic-anti-doping-between-the-1960s-and-the# (accessed 26 May 2017)

156 Sean Ingle (n 134)

157 CAS 2007/A/1416

National and the International Federation. To start with, Scherf, an American athlete, was at the time of the dispute a student at Harvard University. She thus had access to a variety of resources in arguing her case.

Scherf was "diagnosed with exercise induced asthma"[158] in 2003 and accordingly applied for and was granted a TUE by her national anti-doping organization for the year 2006 and 2007. Scherf received the TUE from her International Federation only for the year 2005.[159] Hence, she was a beneficiary of the TUE system and did not face any problem in getting the TUE, continuously, for three years. The problem arose only because she, as well as her national anti-doping organization, were confused as to the scope of her TUE because in 2007 Scherf's TUE was only good for national and other non-international athletic competitions. For international competitions she had to apply for a TUE with her International Federation viz. the IAAF. Considering her background, as well as the fact that her national anti-doping organization viz. the United States Anti-Doping Agency (USADA) was one of the most proactive anti-doping organizations, the confusion was surprising. Scherf was nonetheless unsure as to her status, since she was planning to participate in the 2007 Gold Coast Marathon in Australia.[160] The USADA believed that for this marathon Scherf needed an IAAF TUE. Both the athlete as well her anti-doping organization diligently followed up the TUE application process with the IAAF. However, the TUE decision was delayed and their wait prolonged. As the date of the Gold Coast Marathon neared, Scherf became desperate. The USADA then advised her to check with the marathon organizer as to the likelihood of drug testing. The strategy was that Scherf would not participate if there was to be drug testing. Somehow, she got the impression that in all probability there would be no drug testing.[161] Here the role of USADA is to be noted. During the proceedings before the CAS, it was established that the IAAF had, in 2007, published a list of events that did not recognize the Gold Coast Marathon as an international event.[162] This meant that Scherf's TUE, issued by the USADA, was good enough for the Gold Coast Marathon, since it would be a non-international event.

The USADA was unaware of the IAAF notification, adding to the athlete's confusion. Here one is forced to reflect on the plight of a non-elite/developing country athlete, who is not privileged with the advantages of being in a First World country. Further, their anti-doping organizations are far behind the USADA in terms of advocacy or outreach programmes. If Scherf's confusion was, to a large extent, contributed to by the USADA, a non-elite athlete has far more reasons to complain. Due to the USADA's ignorance/negligence, Scherf participated in the marathon, under the belief that she did not have a

---

158 Ibid para 2.2
159 Ibid
160 Ibid para 2.4
161 Ibid para 2.10, 2.11, 2.12
162 Ibid para 2.16

legitimate TUE. Consequently, when she was required to undergo drug test-ing at the end of the race she panicked and refused to submit for drug testing. She panicked because she believed that in the absence of the TUE her use of asthma drugs amounted to an ADRV.[163] Unfortunately, refusing to submit to a drug test amounts to an ADRV.[164] She took the chance on her father's advice because he felt that Scherf would face a lesser penalty for a missing drug test than testing positive for a banned drug.[165] Here the role of the IAAF was also problematic. The IAAF delayed the process of approving the TUE.[166] Further, there is no indication that the IAAF had widely publicized the new list of international competitions. Against such a background the ignorance and confusion of the athlete are understandable. Interestingly, the current ISTUE requires the TUEC to give a decision within twenty-one days from receipt of the complete TUE application. However, there are no consequences for the TUEC or anti-doping organization in case of delay. In the context of develop-ing/non-elite perspective the time frame does not amount to much as there is no recourse to any remedy or compensation provision against the entity that has contributed to the delay. Thus, Scherf's case flags the grey area of the TUE process from a non-elite perspective. The loopholes and the errors of the anti-doping organizations as well as the International Federations, makes the non-elite's position vulnerable and creates barriers to accessing the TUE itself.

The next case points to the other problem that a non-elite/developing country athlete is likely to face in the context of a TUE. In *Mr Robert Berger v. World Anti-Doping Authority*,[167] the athlete, who was a shooter, was challenging the rejection of his TUE application. The athlete was suffering from chronic heart disease for which he needed to take metoprolol, a beta-blocker. In the sport of shooting, beta-blockers are prohibited, both in and out of competition, by WADA.[168] Hence, the only way he could have continued the usage of the medi-cine as well as compete in sports was through the TUE. Unfortunately for the athlete, his International Federation viz. the International Paralympic Com-mittee (IPC) rejected the TUE application.[169] On the athlete's application to WADA for review, WADA did not reverse the IPC TUEC's decision.[170] That led the athlete to approach the CAS. The IPC TUEC's reasoning was exclusively

---

163 Ibid para 2.14
164 Ibid para 2.15. See World Anti-Doping Agency (n 16), Article 2.3 [Evading, Refusing or Failing to Submit to Sample Collection Evading Sample collection, or without compelling justification, refusing or failing to submit to Sample collection after notification as authorized in applicable anti-doping rules.]
165 CAS 2007/A/1416 (n 157)
166 Ibid para 2.7
167 CAS 2009/A/1948
168 Ibid para 1
169 Ibid para 6
170 Ibid para 7

based on the concern that none of the existing medical and scientific evidence could decisively prove the lack of performance-enhancing effects of the beta-blocker.[171] Understandably then the athlete had to counter this finding before the CAS, since the WADA also went along with the IPC TUEC.[172] There was the preliminary issue of interpreting Article 13.4 of the 2009 WADA Code. Article 13.4 of the 2009 Code allowed appeal to CAS against WADA TUEC only if it reversed the decision of the anti-doping organization. In the case of non-reversal, appeal to the CAS could only be against the decision of the anti-doping organization TUEC.[173] The decision of WADA not to reverse the decision of the anti-doping organization TUEC could not be appealed. In this case, the athlete had filed the appeal to the CAS against WADA for not reversing the IPC TUEC's decision. This was not covered by Article 13.4 of the 2009 Code.[174] Hence, the CAS had no jurisdiction in the matter. Nonetheless, the CAS proceeded with the matter based "upon the express jurisdiction conferred . . . by the parties to this Appeal."[175] The 2015 Code has done away with the confusion and ambiguity that afflicted Article 13.4. The current article reads as "TUE decisions may be appealed exclusively as provided in Article 4.4."[176] As per Article 4.4 non-reversal of the anti-doping organization TUEC's decision by the WADA TUEC, appeal to the CAS lies only against the anti-doping organization TUEC's decision.[177]

Having thus sorted the issue of jurisdiction, the CAS went on to evaluate the medical evidence and the expert witness produced by Berger. The athlete tried to prove that the use of beta-blocker did not have performance-enhancing effects. CAS perused through the conflicting scientific evidence both against and in favour of the athlete. The CAS reasoned that the WADA TUEC had relied on

---

171 Ibid para 12
172 Ibid para 18
173 WADA Code 2009, Article 13.4 [Decisions by WADA reversing the grant or denial of a therapeutic use exemption may be appealed exclusively to CAS by the Athlete or the Anti-Doping Organization whose decision was reversed. Decisions by Anti-Doping Organizations other than WADA denying therapeutic use exemptions, which are not reversed by WADA, may be appealed by International Level Athletes to CAS and by other Athletes to the national-level reviewing body described in Article 13.2.2. If the national-level reviewing body reverses the decision to deny a therapeutic use exemption, that decision may be appealed to CAS by WADA. When an Anti-Doping Organization fails to take action on a properly submitted therapeutic use exemption application within a reasonable time, the Anti-Doping Organization's failure to decide may be considered a denial for purposes of the appeal rights provided in this Article.]
174 CAS 2009/A/1948 (n 167) para 41
175 Ibid para 69
176 Code 2015, Article 13.4
177 Ibid, Article 4.4.7 [Any TUE decision by an International Federation (or by a National Anti-Doping Organization where it has agreed to consider the application on behalf of an International Federation) that is not reviewed by Wada, or that is reviewed by Wada but is not reversed upon review, may be appealed by the athlete and/or the athlete's national anti-doping organization, exclusively to CAS.]

the most relevant scientific data and studies which clearly prove the performance enhancing effect of beta-blockers. The CAS inferred that

> even though Mr Berger's heart rate, as the Holter monitoring tests revealed, ranged still at high levels notwithstanding his ingestion of metoprolol, an improved shooting performance, even if not due to changes in cardiovascular variables such as changes in heart rate, could, indeed will likely, be the result of a reduced neural hand tremor as the study at the University of Copenhagen concludes. This information, in the minds of the WADA TUEC, was entirely relevant.[178]

This conclusion on the part of the CAS begs one to question how, with Berger's kind of heart condition, will he ever get a TUE? Further, how will he be able to prove the lack of performance enhancement? Importantly, with a critical heart condition that is stabilized by the use of beta-blockers, how can any TUEC decide what would be more than a normal state of health for such athletes? WADA, in its guidelines on medical information to support the TUEC's decisions, has accepted that "[s]ince a number of athletes requiring Beta-blocker therapy for one of the abovementioned conditions might be significantly ill and impaired, defining the 'state of normal health' in these cases represents a further challenge."[179] The CAS clearly failed to emphasize the TUEC's need to individualize the process. An athlete's condition measured without the use of the prohibited substance needs to be evaluated. The difficulty is, as in the case of Berger, that stoppage of the medicine would be life-threatening. Ironically, both the IPC TUEC as well as the WADA TUEC accepted that the beta-blocker was necessary to treat the athlete's condition and that there were no viable alternatives. In such a situation rejecting it on the grounds of perceived performance enhancement is problematic. And that adds to the problem of TUEs themselves, because there is no clarity on the method of determining the performance-enhancing effect. There are no objective criteria against which the condition of the affected athlete can be judged. For non-elite/developing country athletes the countering of scientific evidence relied upon by TUEC will be much more difficult in the absence of resources. As noted, proving the absence of performance enhancement is that much more difficult since one has no idea how to go about it. It takes us back to the question with which the discussion on TUE started viz. what is normal?

International Shooting Sport Federation (ISSF) v. World Anti-Doping Agency (WADA)[180] further highlights the difficulties of TUEs. Here, too, the athlete,

178 CAS 2009/A/1948 (n 167) para 114
179 World Anti-Doping Agency, "TUE Physician Guidelines Medical Information to Support the Decisions of TUECs- Cardiovascular Conditions: The Therapeutic Use of Beta-blockers in Athletes" (December 2015) www.wada-ama.org/sites/default/files/resources/files/wada-tpg-cardiovascular_conditions-1.1.pdf (accessed 12 May 2017)
180 Arbitration CAS 2013/A/3437

seventeen-year-old Nadine Ungerank, a shooter, was diagnosed with a cardiac problem. She was prescribed atenolol, a beta-blocker.[181] Being on the Prohibited List, the athlete applied to her NADO for TUE, and the same was granted.[182] She was required to have a TUE from her International Federation viz. International Shooting Sport Federation (ISSF) for the purpose of participating in international competitions. She failed to apply for the same and participated in the European Shooting Confederation's 10 Meter Air Rifle Championship in Odense, Denmark[183] without the ISSF TUE. On being tested, she returned a positive result, and the ISSF proceeded against her for an ADRV.[184] However, she was imposed with a reduced sanction period of three months.[185] Later she applied for an ISSF TUE but the same was rejected by the ISSF TUEC.[186] The main thrust of the decision was (1) failure of the athlete to prove the absence of a performance-enhancing effect and (2) failure of the athlete to prove lack of alternative treatment.[187] The ISSF TUEC reiterated that compliance with all the requirements of the ISTUE was mandatory. The athlete then applied to WADA for review of this decision. The WADA TUEC reversed the ISSF TUEC decision and directed that the athlete be granted the TUE.[188] The said decision was based on the following: (1) the use of the medicine and the treatment were necessary for the health of the athlete; (2) there was no relevant scientific evidence or studies to prove "any distinct capacity of beta-blockers to enhance performance in shooting, there is no evidence-based justification for a categorical prohibition of these substances";[189] (3) there was a lack of therapeutic alternatives; and (4) there was no proof that the "clinical condition requiring treatment has occurred as a consequence of the use of other prohibited substances or methods."[190] In conclusion, the WADA TUEC decided that denial of the TUE to the athlete would be wrong since the same would be "based on a speculated, but entirely unproven, positive benefit of beta-blockers on shooting performance."[191]

This decision of the WADA TUEC is in contrast to the approach of the WADA TUEC in Berger's case.[192] In that case the WADA TUEC held that "Considering the numerous publications in the scientific literature suggesting a significant improvement of sports performance and activities requiring precision and accuracy, such as shooting, by the use of different betablocking agents.

181 Ibid para 5
182 Ibid para 7–8
183 Ibid para 9
184 Ibid para 12
185 Ibid
186 Ibid para 17
187 Ibid para 18
188 Ibid para 20
189 Ibid
190 Ibid
191 Ibid
192 CAS 2009/A/1948 (n 167)

In these studies, it was demonstrated that shooting skills were significantly improved."[193] In contrast, the WADA TUEC in the ISSF case[194] dismissed the literature relied upon by the ISSF TUEC by stating that the studies "did not show any relationship between the cardiovascular effects of the beta-blockers and the shooting scores." Interestingly, the WADA TUEC in this case notes, based on one study, that "there might be hyper-responders to beta-blockers in whom the heart rate response is so blunted as to impair performance and that some level of anxiety (as manifested by an increase in heart rate) is important for performance. The authors identified the need for further studies to assess these individual effects."[195] Evidently then there are contrasting approaches amongst the WADA TUEC itself giving ambiguous signals to all anti-doping organizations. On one hand, the beta-blockers are regarded as having a performance-enhancing effect, and on the other hand it is advised to treat each beta-blocker TUE case carefully. One approach relies on scientific literature and studies as the ultimate proof, the other dismisses the literature, amongst others, based on conflicting findings. From a non-elite/developing country athlete perspective this ambiguity adds to the confusion and complicates the TUE application process itself. On the other hand, the ISSF did follow a similar approach as that of the IPC in the Berger case.[196] Hence, the ISSF was not happy with the reversal of its decision by the WADA TUEC. Accordingly, an appeal was filed with the CAS. The CAS looked into the WADA TUEC's argument pertaining to lack of scientific evidence on the performance-enhancing effect of beta-blockers. Based on the WADA TUEC's deliberations, the CAS was not convinced that beta-blockers have a remote possibility of having a performance-enhancing effect in cases of therapeutic use. Further, the CAS did not agree with the WADA TUEC that "the scientific literature suggests only 'a remote possibility'"[197] of performance-enhancing effect of beta-blockers. To substantiate this point, the CAS referred to the fact that all beta-blockers are included on the WADA Prohibited List. Importantly, as the CAS points out, they are banned for shooting both in and out of competition.[198]

This analyses led the CAS to question the very premise of the WADA TUEC decision viz. absence of proof of the performance-enhancing effect of beta-blockers in cases of therapeutic use. The next point on which the CAS rejected the WADA TUEC's decision was the effect of the beta-blocker on the athlete viz. Nadine Ungerank. The WADA TUEC had compared the athlete's performance, pre and post atenolol usage, with that of another athlete of similar age. This methodology of the WADA TUEC to prove the lack of a performance-enhancement

193 Ibid para 89
194 Arbitration CAS 2013/A/3437 (n 180)
195 Ibid para 20
196 CAS 2009/A/1948 (n 167)
197 Ibid para 310
198 Ibid para 312

effect in Ungerank was challenged and rejected by the CAS. The CAS pointed out that

> no reliance can be placed on a single comparator about whom nothing is known other than she was also female, an elite shooter, and had agreed mean scores between the ages of 12–18 in air rifle and 50 metre 3 position shooting. It is not necessary to be a statistician to recognise that as a comparator such single sample is manifestly inadequate. At the very least the records of a cohort of similarly circumstanced competitors at the same competitions as the Athlete would have been required to draw any sensible conclusions.[199]

The other flaw in the WADA TUEC methodology, as pointed out by the CAS, was its reliance on the athlete's performance statistics. The CAS reasoned that the time period for which the performances of the athlete was taken was inadequate. The CAS concluded that

> this is a too short time perspective on which to rely. If from the material provided one chooses all competitions before and after the starting of the treatment one can recognise an increase in the average scores after the commencement of the Atenolol treatment. While such increase may be what one would expect in the case of an Athlete when she/he is both maturing and on receipt of better training and other benefits, the influence of Atenolol cannot be discounted.[200]

During the proceedings before the CAS, WADA provided the complete result sheet detailing the performances of the athlete. The period covered was from 2009 to 2011. The CAS, after analysing the data, concluded that *"if one compares the scoring between the years one can observe that the scores accomplished after the start of the treatment with atenolol are the best whether the comparison is of average score, lowest score or highest score."*[201] The CAS further emphasized that the burden is on the athlete to prove *"whether this progress and the excellent competitive results is a function of physical development, better training, better equipment or the impact of atenolol?"*[202] Unfortunately for the athlete, the CAS was not convinced that the evidence was good enough to prove the lack of performance-enhancing effect on the athlete.

The most crucial point in the CAS award is that nowhere did it doubt the inability of the athlete to discharge the burden proof viz. balance of probability. The CAS though found the evidence adduced not convincing enough to negate allusions to performance-enhancing effect of atenolol. The crucial point then,

199 Arbitration CAS 2013/A/3437 (n 180) para 316
200 Ibid para 319
201 Ibid para 322
202 Ibid para 323

what more should the athlete do? The CAS concluded its analysis by declaring that "while all human rights instruments recognize that there is a right to life, none recognize that there is an equivalent right to sport."[203] This view of the CAS contradicts the fourth principle of Olympism, as enshrined in the Olympic Charter. The fourth principle of Olympism very clearly states that "[t]he practice of sport is a human right. Every individual must have the possibility of practising sport, without discrimination of any kind and in the Olympic spirit, which requires mutual understanding with a spirit of friendship, solidarity and fair play."[204] This contradiction adds to the problem of the athletes in general and non-elite/developing country athletes in particular in their attempts to seek TUEs. The CAS's dismissal of right to sport has a telling effect since it renders getting a TUE nearly impossible. Further, it also leads one to question the kinds of evidence that elite athletes like Simone Biles or Serena Williams are able to provide that is good enough to convince their International Federations to grant them TUEs. The recent leak of their medical documents clearly shows that they have been granted TUEs without much ado. For example, the leaked documents showed that Simone Biles had been granted a TUE from 2012 extending up to 2018.[205]

A reading of the WADA document relating to the medical information needed to support attention-deficit/hyperactivity disorder (ADHD) shows that the TUE for this condition can be granted for up to four years at a time.[206] So the duration of the TUE for Biles for ADHD is indicative of the laxity of the system. Further, the CAS's decisions in the beta-blocker TUE cases, as discussed above, also proves that some TUEs are almost impossible to be availed of while others are far more randomly granted. The case comment by WADA on the CAS decision in the beta-blocker TUE cases affirms the uncertainty. WADA notes that

> CAS has considerably limited an athlete's prospect of obtaining a TUE for Beta-blockers. This is mainly due to the high standard of proof that an athlete must satisfy to demonstrate that they derive no individual performance enhancement from their use. Indeed, without specifically answering the

203 Ibid para 327
204 Olympic Charter, "Fundamental Principles of Olympism" https://stillmed.olympic.org/media/Document%20Library/OlympicOrg/General/EN-Olympic-Charter.pdf#_ga=2.146302775.2066783038.1497077375-1924997101.1497077375 (accessed 29 May 2017)
205 Andrew McGarry, "WADA Hack Highlights Use of Banned Substances in Sport Through Therapeutic Use Exemptions" ABC News (New York, 14 September 2016) www.abc.net.au/news/2016-09-14/wada-hack-the-latest-chapter-in-the-weaponising-of-world-sport/7843166 (accessed 29 May 2017)
206 World Anti-Doping Agency, "Medical Information to Support the Decisions of TUE Committees Attention Deficit Hyperactivity Disorder (ADHD) in Children and Adults" (2014) www.wada-ama.org/sites/default/files/resources/files/WADA-MI-ADHD-5.0.pdf (accessed 29 May 2017)

question as to what standard of proof an athlete must satisfy, these CAS decisions effectively apply a standard that is quite close to 'beyond a reasonable doubt.[207]

This sort of jurisprudential ambiguity also adds to the problem of non-elite/developing country athletes. Thus, in the context of getting a TUE the present system is (1) ambiguous, (2) discriminatory, (3) costly and (4) elitist. It's a no-win situation for the non-elites/developing country athletes. And the last point which one could have used to argue the non-existence of an ADRV also establishes the elitist orientation of WADA. As mentioned, the athletes can escape the claim of an ADRV by proving the absence of cause of action. So far the discussion has covered two important grounds that are used to nullify the claim of an ADRV. The first was the validity of the sample test and the second was the TUE. As seen above, the chance of success in case of both the grounds is nearly impossible and gives rise to more questions than answers. The complicated process involved in proving the existence of these grounds is sufficient to discourage the non-elite/developing country athlete. This also means that the hope of nullifying an ADRV is bleak for the non-elite/developing country athlete. Further. the difficulties of proving the two grounds discussed above threatens to tighten the grip of strict liability doctrine. The rigours of the doctrine are further accentuated and an athlete is virtually left with no relief. It is against such a situation that the last ground pertaining to decision limits needs to be analysed. The ensuing discussion will detail out the effectiveness of the ground as well as its current status. The thrust of the discussion will be the cost entailed in challenging the decision limits, as well as the response of the governing bodies/anti-doping organizations to such a challenge. The focus will be on WADA's response to this challenge and the follow-up steps.

Decision limits and the non-elite athlete: chasing an illusion

Decision Limits (DL) are set to determine the threshold that is used to justify the AAF. This means that to nullify the claim of an ADRV one has to challenge the validity of the DL itself. Since the DL is set by WADA, challenging DL means questioning the legitimacy of the method used by the anti-doping organization to prove the ADRV.[208] Till the recent past, there have been cases where DL challenges have been made to disprove an ADRV. The cases, as will be discussed, highlight the efforts needed to challenge DL. Further, the profile of the athletes challenging DL proves that such a challenge could be made exclusively by an elite

207 World Anti-Doping Agency (n 179) 16
208 WADA Technical Document – TD2017DL, "Decision Limits for the Confirmatory Quantification of Threshold Substances" (2017) www.wada-ama.org/sites/default/files/resources/files/2016-12-13_td2017dl.pdf (accessed 10 June 2017)

athlete. A non-elite/developing country athlete will find it extremely difficult to counter the technicalities that are inherent in such a challenge. Further the nuanced arguments required to rebut the scientific data would require an expert witness and reliable literature. The same problem that is seen in the context of the other grounds used for rebutting ADRVs thus bogs down a non-elite/developing country athlete. The first case in which a challenge to DL was made is *Andrus Veerpalu*.[209] An AAF was claimed against the athlete for out-of-competition use of recombinant or exogenous human growth hormone (recGH).[210] RecGH is a type of human growth hormone (hGH)[211] that is on WADA's Prohibited List both in and out of competition.[212]

As soon as the AAF was declared the athlete's National Federation viz. Estonian Ski Association (NSA EST) informed his International Federation viz. Fédération International de Ski (FIS) about his proposed retirement from professional cross-country skiing.[213] Since the AAF was based on A sample testing, the B sample had yet to be tested to affirm the A sample finding. As a result of the talks of retirement, the NSA EST requested postponement of opening of the B sample.[214] Accordingly, the opening of the B sample was delayed. Thereafter, accusations were made by the FIS that the athlete had admitted to the use of recGH and hence he had waived his right to get the B sample opened. Both the athlete and NSA EST vehemently denied the same and requested the opening of the B sample.[215] The B sample analysis confirmed the finding of an AAF. Thus, the FIS got the cause to proceed against the athlete for an ADRV.[216] Herein the case needs to be understood in its proper perspective. The confirmation of an AAF by both the A and B samples *prima facie* proves an ADRV. The only way the athlete could have traditionally challenged the ADRV was by demolishing the validity of tests or by showing TUE. There was in this case no TUE. So the only option was to challenge the tests. However, in this case the athlete went even further and challenged the DL. This was possible if one analysed the background of the athlete.

Andrus Veerpalu is regarded as the most successful Estonian skier as well as one of the strongest classical skiers.[217] Hence, the athlete was comfortably in the posi-

---

209 CAS 2011/A/2566 Andrus Veerpalu v. International Ski Federation

210 Ibid para 6

211 See Human growth hormone (hGH) Testing www.wada-ama.org/en/questions-answers/human-growth-hormone-hgh-testing (Explains the effect of hGH on athletes) (accessed 1 June 2017)

212 Prohibited List-January 2018, S2.3 www.wada-ama.org/sites/default/files/prohibited_list_2018_en.pdf (accessed 1 June 2018)

213 CAS 2011/A/2566 (n 209) para 8

214 Ibid

215 Ibid para 10

216 Ibid para 12

217 SR/OLYMPIC Sports, Andrus Veerpalu www.sports-reference.com/olympics/athletes/ve/andrus-veerpalu-1.html (accessed 14 June 2017)

tion to take on WADA and challenge the validity of the DL. Further, this was the most effective way to counter the claim of an ADRV because it challenged the very basis of the AAF. Hence, when the FIS Doping Panel imposed sanctions on Veerpalu, he challenged the same in an appeal before the CAS. The arguments he took before the FIS Panel and the CAS were on similar lines:

> the [t]est is defective and scientifically invalid, particularly because of unreliable decision limits; second, the Laboratory was not accredited to perform the Test; third, the Test was improperly applied and administered by the DCO and the Laboratory; and fourth, the Athlete's individual circumstances render any positive Test result meaningless. Moreover, the Appellant also denies having admitted to hGH use.[218]

The CAS addressed the DL issue at the end. It first dealt with the athlete's claim of deviation from the ISL. The CAS dismissed the same by concluding that "the Appellant has not demonstrated that any shortcomings or violations of the ISL in the pre-analytical handling, alleged or otherwise, could have led to a false positive finding."[219] The next issue related to the athlete's claim that his individual circumstances led to the AAF. He blamed the high hGH levels on intense physical exercise at high altitude as well as his genetic peculiarity.[220] Understandably the CAS rejected this argument as frivolous, stating that "the Appellant's arguments failed to convince the Panel that any relevant individual circumstances existed, and even if they did, the Appellant failed to demonstrate to the required standard of proof that such individual circumstances could have caused the AAF."[221]

The CAS also upheld the reliability of the tests used to detect recGH in blood samples.[222] As WADA explained,

> [the] testing method is essentially based on the established principle that the normal composition of hGH in blood is a mixture of different isoforms, present at constant relative proportions. In contrast, recGH is comprised almost exclusively of monomeric 22-KDa molecular form. The administration of exogenous recGH not only leads to an increase in the concentration of the 22-KDa isoform but also causes a reduction of the non-22-kDa concentrations, thus altering the natural ratios established between these hGH isoforms.[223]

---

218 CAS 2011/A/2566 (n 209) para 81
219 Ibid para 137
220 Ibid para 138
221 Ibid para 148
222 Ibid para 175
223 See World Anti-Doping Agency, "World Anti-Doping Programme Guidelines hGH Isoform Differential Immunoassays for Anti-Doping Analyses" (June 2014) www.wada-ama.org/sites/

The CAS was convinced that "the hGH Test is a reliable testing method for hGH abuse in professional sports that is based on scientifically correct assumptions and methods. . . . It follows that the Appellant's arguments on the Reliability of the Test are rejected in their entirety."[224] Having thus rejected almost all the arguments of the athlete, the next logical step was to reject the appeal. It is at this stage that the DL challenge comes to the athlete's rescue. The athlete argued that the DL was set too low to include even natural hGH. This would lead to false positives.[225] The athlete further argued that the data used to set the DL was inadequate and excluded relevant samples.[226]

The CAS agreed with the athlete's argument that "the decision limits are over inclusive and could lead to an excessive amount of false positive results."[227] The CAS also agreed with the athlete's argument about the unreliability of the sample used to set the DL. Rejecting the DL set by WADA, the CAS concluded that:

1   "For the purposes of any further studies for determining decision limits for prohibited substances that can be produced endogenously, the Panel recommends that any exclusion of samples from the reference population data be separately documented with reasoning."[228]

2   "[T]he Panel is not comfortably satisfied that the sizes of the samples used were sufficiently large to permit an estimation of the 99.99% point that is sufficiently reliable."[229]

3   "[T]he Panel is of the view that the Respondent has provided insufficient explanations and details about the way in which the decision limits were calculated, to such an extent that the Panel cannot comfortably conclude that they are reliable."[230]

The CAS then had to overrule the finding of the ADRV.[231] From a non-elite/developing country perspective, the case leads to the following conclusions: (1) an athlete may be guilty of an ADRV but can get away by exploiting technical flaws within the anti-doping regime; (2) to exploit the technical loopholes one has to have access to brilliant scientists and experts; (3) failure to challenge the reliability of the tests does not rule out challenging the threshold set for AAF; (4) questioning the threshold and other finer aspects of the testing procedure is

default/files/resources/files/WADA-Guidelines-for-hGH-Differential-Immunoassays-v2.1-2014-EN.pdf (accessed 14 June 2017)
224 CAS 2011/A/2566 (n 209) para 183
225 Ibid para 195
226 Ibid para 197
227 Ibid para 203
228 Ibid para 204
229 Ibid para 205
230 Ibid para 206
231 Ibid para 234

an act in sophistication and would require an enormous number of resources; and (5) such an outcome would be an impossible dream for a resource starved athlete.

Andrus Veerpalu clearly conned the system by getting away with the use of a prohibited substance.[232] The CAS grudgingly observed that

> [t]he Panel notes that there are many factors in this case which tend to indicate that the Athlete did in fact himself administer exogenous hGH, but that for the reason that the decision limits have not been proven as reliable in the course of this proceeding, the violation of the FIS ADR cannot be upheld on appeal.[233]

This case proves the power of elite athletes to benefit from the WADA Code. It substantiates further the accessibility issue that non-elite/developing country athletes face in rebutting an ADRV. It raises concerns about the elitist nature of the WADA Code.

Nationale Anti-Doping Agentur Deutschland v. Patrick Sinkewitz[234] is the next case on DL challenges. Sinkewitz was a professional cyclist, competing at the highest level of the sport. The interesting bit is that he was a serial doper. His first ADRV was in 2007 for usage of a cocktail of prohibited substance viz. testosterone ointment, erythropoietin ("EPO") and blood transfusions.[235] His second ADRV was in 2011 for usage of recGH.[236] This time, however, he successfully challenged the ADRV before the National Arbitral Tribunal (DIS) by proving that "the calculation of the DL for the rec/pit ratio found in the Athlete's samples was not sufficiently documented."[237] This was again a case of an athlete trying to escape the consequences of an ADRV by exploiting the loopholes in the WADA Code. Nonetheless, the National Anti-Doping Agency (NADA) appealed to the CAS.[238] It also requested that the results of the DL review process undertaken by WADA be admitted as new evidence.[239] WADA had undertaken the DL review in view of the *Veerpalu*[240] decision. The CAS decided to hear the new evidence and the experts who had undertaken the review.[241]

Before the CAS the athlete argued on familiar lines challenging the reliability of DL by claiming that the data used for setting the limits "were incomplete and have been unsystematically collected and, in any case, not in accordance

---

232 Chelsea Little, "How WADA Dropped the Ball on the Veerpalu Doping Case" (2013) http://fasterskier.com/fsarticle/how-wada-dropped-the-ball-on-the-veerpalu-doping-case/ (accessed 16 June 2017)
233 CAS 2011/A/2566 (n 209) para 234
234 CAS 2012/A/2857
235 Ibid para 5
236 Ibid para 7
237 Ibid para 17
238 Ibid para 19
239 Ibid para 38
240 CAS 2011/A/2566 (n 209)
241 CAS 2012/A/2857 (n 237) para 137

with the standard of 'good scientific practice'."[242] Further, the data excluded factors such as "ethnicity, physical exercise, sport discipline practiced, time of the sample collection and age, may have an influence on the hGH ratio."[243] Accordingly, there were high chances of false positives. Further, the "DL should have been set at a significantly higher level."[244] Thus, the DL set by WADA could not conclusively prove use of recGH.[245] In light of the ongoing debate on DL, as evident from the Veerpalu case, the CAS ascertained the legal status of DL. At the time of this dispute, DL were only part of the hGH guidelines and hence were not mandatory. Accordingly, DL per se does not lead to a finding of an ADRV. In view of this, the setting of threshold and using the same to declare an AAF and subsequently an ADRV was legally questionable. As the CAS rightly stated, "The hGH Guidelines, including the DL contained in it, are not mandatory but rather a mere recommendation addressed to the WADA accredited laboratories. The DL are not legally binding as such and, therefore, do not legally constitute what an ADRV is."[246] This also meant that a result below the DL might also be the result of doping, since the DL itself had no mandatory effect. The consequence being that since labs are to report only results above DL, they can conveniently ignore the results below DL. So, one could continue to dope ensuring that the ratios are below the DL.

In the context of the case however, CAS used this point to reject the athlete's argument pertaining to the ADRV. The CAS argued that proof of an ADRV is not dependent on the reliability of DL since DL had no legal force.[247] This statement reflects the inconsistencies in the CAS's position on DL challenges. In Veerpalu,[248] the CAS specifically pointed to the unreliability of the DL for rejecting the AAF and the consequent ADRV.[249] Such contradictions raise questions on the reliability as well as uniformity within the anti-doping programme. Interestingly, the CAS concurred with Veerpalu[250] in upholding the validity of the hGH test. It distinguished between analyses of the samples using the hGH test versus interpretation of the test result using DL. The CAS emphasized that the analyses of the sample were done properly, and hence were not to be challenged. DL, however, merely indicate whether the results could be used to report an AAF. This is clearly confusing since without interpretation the test results are meaningless because an AAF is the outcome of interpretation of the test result. This also goes against the Veerpalu[251] decision because

242 Ibid para 187
243 Ibid
244 Ibid
245 Ibid
246 Ibid para 192
247 Ibid para 193
248 CAS 2011/A/2566 (n 209)
249 Ibid para 234
250 Ibid
251 Ibid

in that case the DL was regarded as an integrated aspect of the hGH test. The CAS in that case clearly stated that *"the decision limits determine whether the recGH/pitGH ratios in Kit 1 and Kit 2 qualify as an AAF."*[252] Continuing with this reasoning, the CAS further added to the ambiguity on DL by declaring that "the findings in . . . the Veerpalu award . . . do not undermine the reliability of the DL as such and do not prevent the Panel from taking into consideration the ratios found in the Respondent's samples as a means of evidence."[253] This again is a contradiction because, as pointed out above, the CAS itself insisted that the DL was "not a mandatory precondition in order to prove that the ratios found on the Respondent's samples show the presence of exogenous rec hGH."[254]

The CAS goes on to hold that in view of the higher ratios found in the athlete's sample, the validity or invalidity of the DL has no bearing on the outcome. Accordingly, the *Veerpalu*[255] case was distinguished as that of a "borderline situation which might trigger the benefit of uncertainty for the Athlete."[256] The reasoning gives an impression that the CAS was at the same point in time approbating and reprobating DL. The CAS in this case stated that *Veerpalu*[257] does not declare the DL set by WADA as being unreliable but that "the reliability of the determination of the DL was not sufficiently proven before the respective panels."[258] This play of words does not represent the true picture, because as stated above *Veerpalu*[259] declared the DL set by WADA as unreliable.[260] Thus, on the one hand it rejected DL and on the other hand it tried to justify the DL to treat the ratio in the athlete's sample as proof of an ADRV. The CAS in this case went on to hold that "the ratios found in the Respondent's samples clearly indicate the presence of exogenous recGH and that those elevated ratios cannot be explained by natural sources but only by the administration of recGH."[261] The *Sinkewitz*[262] case thus did not clarify the position on DL. This reaffirms the concerns raised herein about the problems faced by non-elite/developing country athletes. The contradiction in the assessment of similar facts and outcome in a case leads to greater injustice for non-elites because they have to invest far greater in garnering the resources. Hence mistakes and ambiguities within the WADA Code and its interpretation, while detrimental to all athletes in general, marginalizes the non-elites further.

252 Ibid para 184
253 CAS 2012/A/2857 (n 237) para 205
254 Ibid para 193
255 CAS 2011/A/2566 (n 209)
256 CAS 2012/A/2857 (n 234) para 204
257 CAS 2011/A/2566 (n 209)
258 CAS 2012/A/2857 (n 237) para 203
259 CAS 2011/A/2566 (n 209)
260 Ibid para 206
261 CAS 2012/A/2857 (n 237) para 215
262 Ibid

The consequences of WADA's laxity on DL is equally evident in the case of Mr Juha Lallukka.[263] This case also involved a Finnish skier[264] and evaluation of the reliability of the DL set by WADA. Accordingly, the Veerpalu[265] case was the point of reference for both the appellants as well as the respondent.[266] Further, as in the Sinkewitz[267] case, here, too, the domestic adjudicating body went along with the Veerpalu decision and dismissed the claim of ADRV against the athlete.[268] In view of this ruling invalidating DL, WADA appealed to the CAS against the athlete's acquittal. As expected, the athlete's argument proceeded on the basis of the unreliability of DL. As in Sinkewitz,[269] the athlete did not challenge the test or the results nor the ratios found in the sample.[270] He used the Veerpalu[271] decision to substantiate his arguments on DL.[272] Since the Veerpalu case, WADA had undertaken further research on DL and their reliability. In the present case, WADA produced the latest research on DL to prove their reliability.[273] The CAS analysed the same against the specific objections raised in the Veerpalu decision[274] viz. insufficient sample size,[275] unjustified exclusion of certain sample data[276] and uncertainty of the distribution model used.[277] The CAS reasoned that the sample size taken into account for conducting the new studies was "a considerably larger sample than that used for the Initial Study as well as the 2009–2010/2010–2011 Verification Studies, altogether."[278] The CAS also concluded that the new research "described precisely which dataset they used and what samples were included or excluded."[279] Lastly, the CAS concluded that the new findings on DL were based "on new and comprehensive data, and provides a detailed account of the characteristics and properties of the materials and methods used."[280]

The CAS thus accepted that WADA had satisfied its burden of proof (standard of comfortable satisfaction) for proving the reliability of DL through the new findings based on the following factors: "First, the Joint Publication Paper

263 CAS 2014/A/3488 World Anti-Doping Agency v. Mr Juha Lallukka
264 Ibid para 2
265 CAS 2011/A/2566 (n 209)
266 CAS 2014/A/3488 (n 256) para 4
267 CAS 2012/A/2857 (n 237)
268 CAS 2014/A/3488 (n 256) para 23 and 27
269 CAS 2012/A/2857 (n 237)
270 CAS 2014/A/3488 (n 256) para 80
271 CAS 2011/A/2566 (n 209)
272 CAS 2014/A/3488 (n 256) para 81
273 Ibid para 83
274 CAS 2011/A/2566 (n 209)
275 CAS 2014/A/3488 (n 256) para 84–90
276 Ibid para 91–93
277 Ibid para 94–96
278 Ibid para 90
279 Ibid para 92
280 Ibid para 95

on which WADA relies"[281] was prepared by independent experts. "Second, this study is based on a considerable and large dataset"[282] which was peer-reviewed. "Third, the study is said to establish decision limits with a 99.99% specificity."[283] The CAS Panel was "comfortably satisfied that WADA has met its burden of proof" vis-à-vis "the reliability both of its Growth Hormone Test and of the decision limits"[284] as published in the new guideline. In this instance the CAS also relied on the *Sinkewitz*[285] case, in particular the distinction made between DL and test analysis and the non-binding nature of the DL.[286] Accordingly, the CAS took account of the high ratio in the athlete's sample and affirmed it to be a case of an ADRV.[287] This approach thus further propagated the contradiction and ambiguity on DL as seen earlier in the *Sinkewitz* case.[288] For both, the CAS Panel was caught in the dilemma of ignoring the relevance of DL on one hand and relying on the DL to interpret the ratio in the samples on the other hand.

In this case the CAS Panel made another fundamental blunder. It applied comfortable satisfaction as the standard of proof to assess the athlete's evidence. Thus, the CAS held that "the Athlete is not in a position to prove to the comfortable satisfaction of the Panel that external factors may have had an impact on his ratio values, which could have led to a false positive. He has not so proven to the comfortable satisfaction of the Panel."[289] This blatant incorrect application of the WADA-mandated burden of proof is enough to ruin any athlete's career, and more so that of a non-elite/developing country athlete.[290] If the CAS was to accept WADA's new evidence on the reliability of DL, then it ought to do so on sound and settled principles of law. Since the athlete in this case was depending on legal aid from the CAS[291] to fight the case, he understandably did not have the means to challenge the CAS decision before the Swiss Federal Tribunal.[292] The other point which is problematic is the reliance on the new DL published in 2014. Since the cause of action arose in 2011, such reliance amounts to retroactive application of the law.[293] The CAS dismissed such concerns by reiterating that DL are just guidelines and not enforceable.[294] This was a reiteration of the

281 Ibid para 98
282 Ibid
283 Ibid
284 Ibid
285 CAS 2012/A/2857 (n 237)
286 CAS 2014/A/3488 (n 256) para 106
287 Ibid para 109
288 CAS 2012/A/2857 (n 237)
289 CAS 2014/A/3488 (n 256) para 109
290 World Anti-Doping Agency (n 16) Article 3
291 Ibid para 33
292 Court of Arbitration for Sport, Frequently Asked Questions www.tas-cas.org/en/general-information/frequently-asked-questions.html (accessed 12 June 2017)
293 CAS 2014/A/3488 (n 256) para 111
294 Ibid para 114

Sinkewitz case.[295] This also violates the norm of fairness as it leads to the applicability of rules detrimental to athletes. This manner of application of DL to prove ADRVs clearly leaves no option for the athlete. The conclusion of the CAS was to hold that "the analytical values of assay ratios relating to the Athlete's samples reveal the presence of recombinant hGH."[296] Such has been the impact of these diverging viewpoints on DL that WADA has now included DL in the Technical Documents.[297] Further, the Technical Documents on DL have been made mandatory as part of the ISL in the 2015 WADA Code.[298] This does not in any way alleviate the problems faced by the non-elite/developing country athletes.

Conclusion

The above discussion highlights the various aspects of the current anti-doping regime under the WADA Code. The incorporation of strict liability principle in the Code strengthens the cause of the elites more than the non-elite/developing country athletes. The doctrine imposes unrealistic expectations on them in view of the circumstances of a non-elite/developing country athlete. The Code has incorporated provisions to soften the rigour of the doctrine and to develop a modified form of strict liability. However, it has softened the rigour to the extent of giving chances to an athlete to rebut the presumption of an ADRV. On the failure of the athlete to rebut the presumption of an ADRV, the result of the event is automatically disqualified, and the rebuttal is excessively tough since one has to challenge the entire system and the result management process. Alternatively, one has to show TUE, which is equally tough to obtain. Thus, the resources needed to challenge ADRVs are likely to dissuade non-elite/developing country athletes from pursuing the matter. These inbuilt constraints thus tend to make WADA Code an elitist doctrine.

Bibliography

Anderson, Jack, *Modern Sports Law–A Textbook* (Hart Publishing, 2010)

---

295 CAS 2012/A/2857 (n 237)
296 CAS 2014/A/3488 (n 256) para 123
297 WADA Technical Document – TD2017DL, Decision Limits for the Confirmatory Quantification of Threshold Substances (2017) www.wada-ama.org/sites/default/files/resources/files/2016-12-13_td2017dl.pdf (accessed 17 June 2017); WADA Technical Document – TD2017DL, Decision Limits for the Confirmatory Quantification of Threshold Substances (2017) www.wada-ama.org/sites/default/files/resources/files/wada-td2017dl-v2-en_0.pdf (accessed 18 January 2017)
298 World Anti-Doping Agency (n 16) Article 6.4 [Laboratories shall analyze Samples and report results in conformity with the international Standard for Laboratories. To ensure effective testing, the Technical Document referenced at Article 5.4.1 will establish risk assessment-based Sample analysis menus appropriate for particular sports and sport disciplines, and laboratories shall analyze Samples in conformity with those menus. . .]

Anderson, Jack, "Doping, Sport and the Law: Time for Repeal of Prohibition?" (2013) 9 (2) *International Journal of Law in Context* 135

Arbitration CAS 2013/A/3437

Arbitration CAS Anti-Doping Division (OG Rio) AD 16/005

Brown, Andy, "Fancy Bears Hack: 107 Athletes; 23 Countries; 25 Sports" (2016) www.sportsintegrityinitiative.com/fancy-bears-hack-107-athletes-23-countries-25-sports/ (accessed 20 May 2017)

Canadian Center for Ethics in Sports, "Conflict of Interest in Anti-Doping" (2016) http://cces.ca/blog/conflict-interest-anti-doping (accessed 13 April 2017)

CAS 2001/A/317 (2001)

CAS 2007/A/1416

CAS 2009/A/1752 Vadim Devyatovskiy v/ IOC; CAS 2009/A/1753 Ivan Tsikhan v/ IOC

CAS 2009/A/1912 (2009)

CAS 2009/A/1948

CAS 2010/A/2235 (2011)

CAS 2010/A/2235 Union Cycliste Internationale (UCI) v. T. & Olympic Committee of Slovenia (OCS) (2011)

CAS 2011/A/2479 (2011)

CAS 2011/A/2566 Andrus Veerpalu v. International Ski Federation

CAS 2012/A/2857

CAS 2014/A/3759 Dutee Chand v Athletics Federation of India (AFI) & The International Association of Athletics Federations (IAAF)

CAS 94/129

CAS ad hoc Division (OG Rio) 16/023 (2016)

Coe, Sebastian, "We Cannot Move from Strict Liability Rule" *The Telegraph* (London, 5 February 2004) www.telegraph.co.uk/sport/othersports/drugsinsport/2373729/We-cannot-move-from-strict-liability-rule.html

Court of Arbitration for Sport, Frequently Asked Questions www.tas-cas.org/en/general-information/frequently-asked-questions.html (accessed 12 June 2017)

Cox, Neville, "Legalisation of Drug Use in Sport' (2002) 2 *ISLR* 77

Cox, Thomas Wyatt, "The International War Against Doping: Limiting the Collateral Damage from Strict Liability" (2014) *Vanderbilt Journal of Transnational Law*, 47 www.vanderbilt.edu/wp-content/uploads/sites/78/CoxFinalReviewComplete.pdf (accessed 23 April 2017)

David, Paul, A *Guide to the World Anti-Doping Code-the Fight for the Spirit of Sport* (Cambridge University Press, 2017)

du Toit, Niel, "Strict Liability and Sports Doping – What Constitutes a Doping Violations and What Is the Effect Thereof on the Team?" (2011) *International Sports Law Journal*, 163 www.doping.nl/media/kb/2044/20131023T040659-ISLJ_2011_3-4%20-%20163-164%20Niel%20du%20Toit.pdf (accessed 22 April 2017)

Ekwurtzel, Karl, "Why You're Not an Olympian: Athletes Built for Their Sports" *ABC News* (New York, 7 August 2012) http://abcnews.go.com/Sports/olympics/olympic-physiques-michael-phelps-usain-bolt-athletes-built/story?id=16917476 (accessed 15 May 2017)

Fancy Bears' Hack Team, "American Athletes Caught Doping 2016–09–13" https://fancybear.net/pages/1.html (accessed 15 May 2017)

Fitzpatrick, Ben, "Strict Liability: Importation Offence" (2004) 68 (3) *Journal of Criminal Law* 195

Hard, Matthew, "Caught in the Net: Athletes' Rights and the World Anti-Doping Agency" (2010) 19 *Southern California Interdisciplinary Law Journal* 533

Human growth hormone (hGH) Testing www.wada-ama.org/en/questions-answers/human-growth-hormone-hgh-testing (Explains the effect of hGH on athletes) (accessed 1 June 2017)

Ingle, Sean, "Wada Hacking Scandal: Debate Turns to the Use of Powerful Legal Drugs-condemnation of Hackers Is Followed by Questions Regarding the Processes of Applying for and Taking Certain Therapeutic Remedies" *The Guardian* (London, 15 September 2016) www.theguardian.com/sport/2016/sep/14/wada-hacking-abuse-debate-theraputic-use-drugs (accessed 21 May 2017)

International Council of Arbitration for Sport, "Guidelines on Legal Aid Before the Court of Arbitration for Sport" (2016) www.tas-cas.org/fileadmin/user_upload/Legal_Aid_Rules_2016_English.pdf (accessed 17 May 2017)

Kaufmann-Kohler, Gabrielle Antonio Rigozzi and Giorgio Malinverni, "Legal Opinion on the Conformity of Certain Provisions of the Draft World Anti-Doping Code with Commonly Accepted Principles of International Law" (2003) www.wada-ama.org/sites/default/files/resources/files/kaufmann-kohler-full.pdf (accessed 3 April 2017)

Kayser, Bengt, Alexander Mauron and Andy Miah, "Current Anti-Doping Policy: A Critical Appraisal" BMC *Medical Ethics*, 2007 https://bmcmedethics.biomedcentral.com/articles/10.1186/1472-6939-8-2 (accessed 19 May 2015)

Little, Chelsea, "How WADA Dropped the Ball on the Veerpalu Doping Case" (2013) http://fasterskier.com/fsarticle/how-wada-dropped-the-ball-on-the-veerpalu-doping-case/ (accessed 16 June 2017)

McCutcheon, Paul, "Sports Discipline, Natural Justice and Strict Liability" (1999) 28 *Anglo-American Law Review* 37

McGarry, Andrew, "WADA Hack Highlights Use of Banned Substances in Sport Through Therapeutic Use Exemptions" ABC *News* (New York, 14 September 2016) www.abc.net.au/news/2016-09-14/wada-hack-the-latest-chapter-in-the-weaponising-of-world-sport/7843166 (accessed 29 May 2017)

McLaren, Richard H. "Athlete Biological Passport: The Juridical Viewpoint" (2012) 4 *ISLR* 77

Mens Tennis Forum, "2015 CIRC Report: Therapeutic Use Exemptions (TUEs) Are Abused" www.menstennisforums.com/2-general-messages/835241-2015-circ-report-therapeutic-use-exemptions-tues-abused.html (accessed 27 May 2017)

Mohney, Gillian, "Simone Biles' ADHD Meds Among Common Drugs Banned from Olympics" ABC *News* (New York, 14 September 2016) http://abcnews.go.com/Health/simone-biles-adhd-meds-common-drugs-banned-olympics/story?id=42081189 (accessed 18 May 2017)

Mulhall, Stephen J. "A Critique of the World Anti-Doping Code" (2006) 64 *Advocate Vancouver* 29

Olympic Charter, "Fundamental Principles of Olympism" https://stillmed.olympic.org/media/Document%20Library/OlympicOrg/General/EN-Olympic-Charter.pdf#_ga=2.146302775.2066783038.1497077375-1924997101.1497077375 (accessed 29 May 2017)

Powell, Jeff, "WADA Appear to Keep Doling Out Therapeutic Use Exemptions Like Sweeties to Children . . . 53 of Our Olympians Were Using Them (and that's just the Brits!)" *Mail Online* (London, 16 September 2016) www.dailymail.co.uk/sport/othersports/article-3792069/WADA-appear-doling-Therapeutic-Use-Exemptions-like-sweeties-children-53-Olympians-using-s-just-Brits.html (accessed 21 May 2017) SR/

Olympic Sports, Andrus Veerpalu www.sports-reference.com/olympics/athletes/ve/andrus-veerpalu-1.html (accessed 14 June 2017)

Procter, Edward, "Dispute Resolution in Sport: The Role of Sport Resolutions (United Kingdom)" (2010) 1 *Comment ISLR* www.sportresolutions.co.uk/uploads/related-documents/Dispute_Resolution_in_Sport_-_The_Role_of_Sport_Resolutions_UK.pdf (accessed 17 May 2017)

Prohibited List-January 2018, S2 3 www.wada-ama.org/sites/default/files/prohibited_list_2018_en.pdf (accessed 1 June 2018)

Queens Bench Division Lexis Nexis Academic (Transcript, Blackwell & Partners, 1988)

Reasoned Decision of the United States Anti-Doping Agency on Disqualification and Ineligibility, United States Anti-Doping Agency, Claimant v. Lance Armstrong, Respondent (2012) https://d3epuodzu3wuis.cloudfront.net/ReasonedDecision.pdf

Reinold, Marcel, "Arguing Against Doping: A Discourse Analytical Study on Olympic Anti-Doping Between the 1960s and the Late 1980s' (7 May 2012) *International Olympic Committee Postgraduate Research Grant Programme 2011 Final Research Report* https://library.olympic.org/Default/doc/SYRACUSE/62313/arguing-against-doping-a-discourse-analytical-study-on-olympic-anti-doping-between-the-1960s-and-the# (accessed 26 May 2017)

Spencer, J. R. "Strict liability and the European Convention" (2004) 63 (1) *Cambridge Law' Journal* 10

Sport, Guardian, "Froome and Wiggins Defend TUEs Use as Team GB Athletes Warned Over Leaks" (London, 15 September 2016) www.theguardian.com/sport/2016/sep/15/chris-froome-defends-use-tues-wada-hacking-leaks (accessed 25 May 2017)

UKHL 37 www.publications.parliament.uk/pa/ld199899/ldjudgmt/jd990722/modahl.htm [1999] (accessed 15 May 2017)

WADA Code 2009, Article 13.4

WADA Technical Document – TD2017DL, "Decision Limits for the Confirmatory Quantification of Threshold Substances" (2017) www.wada-ama.org/sites/default/files/resources/files/2016-12-13_td2017dl.pdf (accessed 10 June 2017)

World Anti-Doping Agency, "Athlete Biological Passport" (2017) www.wada-ama.org/en/athlete-biological-passport (accessed 14 April 2017)

World Anti-Doping Agency, "Athlete Biological Passport Operating Guidelines" (2017) www.wada-ama.org/sites/default/files/resources/files/guidelines_abp_v6_2017_jan_en.pdf (accessed 16 April 2017)

World Anti-Doping Agency, "Medical Information to Support the Decisions of TUE Committees Attention Deficit Hyperactivity Disorder (ADHD) in Children and Adults" (2014) www.wada-ama.org/sites/default/files/resources/files/WADA-MI-ADHD-5.0.pdf (accessed 29 May 2017)

World Anti-Doping Agency, "TUE Physician Guidelines Medical Information to Support the Decisions of TUECs-Cardiovascular Conditions: The Therapeutic Use of Beta-blockers in Athletes" (December 2015) www.wada-ama.org/sites/default/files/resources/files/wada-tpg-cardiovascular_conditions-1.1.pdf (accessed 12 May 2017)

World Anti-Doping Agency, "World Anti-Doping Code" (2015) www.wada-ama.org/sites/default/files/resources/files/wada-2015-world-anti-doping-code.pdf (accessed 27 April 2017)

World Anti-Doping Agency, "World Anti-Doping Program Guidelines hGH Isoform Differential Immunoassays for Anti-Doping Analyses" (June 2014) www.wada-ama.org/sites/default/files/resources/files/WADA-Guidelines-for-hGH-Differential-Immunoassays-v2.1-2014-EN.pdf (accessed 14 June 2017)

World Anti-Doping Agency-play True, "Frequently Asked Questions (FAQ)-Therapeutic Use Exemptions (TUEs)" (17 November 2011) www.wada-ama.org/sites/default/files/resources/files/2016-11-17-qa_tues_en.pdf (accessed 19 May 2017)

World Anti-Doping Agency-play True, "World Anti-Doping Code" (2003) www.wada-ama.org/sites/default/files/resources/files/wada_code_2003_en.pdf (accessed 13 May 2017)

World Anti-Doping Code, "International Standard for Laboratories" (2016) www.wada-ama.org/sites/default/files/resources/files/isl_june_2016.pdf (accessed 1 May 2017)

World Anti-Doping Code, "International Standard for Testing and Investigation [Annex L – Results Management Requirements and Procedures for the Athlete Biological Passport]" (2017) www.wada-ama.org/sites/default/files/resources/files/2016-09-30_-_isti_final_january_2017.pdf (accessed 1 May 2017)

World Anti-Doping Code, "International Standard-Therapeutic Use Exemptions" (2016), Article 4.1 www.wada-ama.org/sites/default/files/resources/files/wada-2016-istue-final-en_0.pdf (accessed 12 May 2017)

Chapter 4

WADA from a non-elite perspective

The missing link in the anti-doping discourse

Introduction

This chapter builds upon the previous chapter, wherein the flaws within the WADA Code are analysed from the perspective of an elitist versus non-elitist debate. In this chapter, the debate is deconstructed further to understand the situation of developing country/non-elite athletes. With the Russian doping scandal looming large, more measures are expected to be taken to detect doping, hence the concern for a developing country/non-elite athlete is immense. Lack of accessibility and education on anti-doping programmes is just one of the many problems. Additionally, the approach of the national sports governing bodies to the concerns of these athletes remains inadequate. The situation prevailing in India best exemplifies the developing country/non-elite athlete's dilemmas. Caught within this web of disinformation and no information, developing country athletes are left to fend for themselves. This lack of support extends right from the day the first pill is inadvertently consumed to the day the arguments are closed before the Court of Arbitration of Sport. The pertinent question then for the policymakers is how to incorporate the narrative of the developing country athlete into the current anti-doping discourse. The existing WADA Code exemplifies homogenization at the cost of dismissing all alternate viewpoints on the topic. In view of the gaping holes that the Russian scandal has brought forth, it's pertinent that other perspectives, outside the existing elite sportsperson's narrative, be taken into account. And this is precisely the argument this chapter tries to articulate.

Non-elite of the sports – identifying the silent group

The non-elite of professional sports are those who are from developing countries and who do not enjoy the spotlight of a star performer. Though the athlete may be successful in terms of medal tally, the athlete is not equal in terms of financial empowerment. Developing country athletes may have the potential and the skill to win competitions, but they do not have the means to access a world-class facility. To the athlete, the adage of Citius Altius Fortius does not apply; the athlete participates not for the sake of winning, but for the sake of earning a livelihood. In a country like India, jobs in government-run institutions like railways, universities, the postal service and so on are available against sports quota.[1] In this scenario, sports become an important source of livelihood and thus limit the choice of the sportsperson. A developing country is identified as"[countries] having a standard of living or level of industrial production well below that possible with financial or technical aid; a country that is not yet highly industrialized."[2] The crunch on resources is the main issue within these countries. Lack of resources means that different sectors of development will be prioritized. When there are hungry mouths to feed and primary education and health programmes to be funded, sports will be one of the last sectors to be prioritized. Against this background the non-elite sportpersons of the world have to deal with a sophisticated anti-doping regulatory system. WADA Code compliance and legal procedures, as referred to in the previous chapter, act as a double whammy. An athlete in the non-elite group of the developing country, usually enters the sports arena with certain inherent disadvantages.

Firstly, the athlete will lack the education needed to understand the implications of doping. Secondly, the athlete will need to understand the differences between permissible and non-permissible drug use. Thirdly, if caught on the wrong side of the WADA system, the athlete will require access to legal, financial and scientific resources to bail them out. Finally, the athlete will need to hope and pray that their domestic federation will act swiftly and fairly in case of any problem vis-à-vis WADA compliance. A major problem is support staff. A vast majority of non-elite developing country athletes will be complete novices in terms of the do's and don'ts of the anti-doping programme. Hence, they are completely dependent on their support staff for all anti-doping information. Thus, unlike an advanced country athlete, who is given the requisite amount of information about the existing anti-doping compliances, a developing country non-elite has no such liberties. To bring home the point, one can compare the efforts of the Australian Sports Anti-Doping Authority (ASADA) in imparting anti-doping awareness and education vis-à-vis the National Anti-Doping Agency of India (NADA)

The ASADA has developed advanced and structured certificate courses on anti-doping. The courses are designed for the target group. Level 1 anti-doping courses are designed for the general public, that is, anyone interested in developing a basic understanding of anti-doping issues. Clearing the assessment designed for a Level 1 course entitles a learner to enroll in Level 2 courses to develop a more advanced understanding of anti-doping issues. Further, there are courses

---

1 Dinesh Prabhu, "Sports Jobs 2019 – Sports Quota Recruitment (16 Govt Vacancies)" *IndGovtJobs* (2018) www.indgovtjobs.in/2014/07/Sports-Quota-Recruitment.html (accessed 5 December 2018)
2 Dictionary.com www.dictionary.com/browse/developing-country (accessed 5 December 2018)

designed specifically for medical practitioners and athlete support personnel, coaches and school athletes. Details of the courses, including modules and assessment plans, are available online. One has to log in to start with any of the courses offered by ASADA.[3]

NADA conducts an anti-doping awareness programme but does not conduct an educational programme. On the NADA website, if one clicks the link titled "[d]etails of Anti-Doping Awareness Programme conducted between April to June 2018"[4] one gets a list. The list provides the addresses of various universities and other institutions where the awareness programme has been conducted. It also provides the dates on which the programme has been conducted. There is no information about the content of the programme nor is there an assessment report on its utility and effectiveness. A visit to NADA's website gives no such information. Additionally, NADA has uploaded anti-doping literature viz. information on the do's and don'ts in few of the different Indian languages. A perusal of the literature gives basic information on the responsibilities of the athlete. There is no booklet on the responsibilities of the athlete support system. There is no information on the chain of authorities that the athlete needs to report to in case of any problems.[5]

Hilariously the website is so poorly managed that when one clicks the link to go to the page on the brand names of PEDs, it goes to the page dealing with publications. This is the case with the Hindi version of the website.[6] Considering that we are talking about accessibility to information, such poor management is telling of the lack of seriousness of NADA in meeting athletes' needs. Insofar as widening the accessibility to NADA and its programmes are concerned, to date no effort has been made to use the online platforms. Barring the uploading of a forty-page document in English, pointing out the different brand names of the PEDs,[7] there is a lack of all social media contact. NADA has not even attempted to upload interactive videos which might help athletes understand the nuances of anti-doping programmes. And one is not yet talking about the decisions given by the NADA Panels. However, the point here is the contrast in approaches to doping enforcement that exist between a developed and a developing country. As Richa Mulchandani shows in her research, the awareness programme conducted by NADA has not resulted in any significant increase in the understanding of anti-doping in sports.[8] One can cite many such issues of structural impediments

3 Australian Government, Australian Anti-Doping Authority https://elearning.asada.gov.au/ (accessed 5 December 2018)

4 NADA, "Anti-Doping Awareness Program Conducted by NADA (April 2018 to June 2018)" www.nadaindia.org/upload_file/document/1532087561.pdf (accessed 5 December 2018)

5 NADA, "Publications" www.nadaindia.org/en/publication-books (accessed 6 December 2018)

6 Visit the Hindi Version www.nadaindia.org/in/publications (accessed 6 December 2018)

7 NADA, "Publications" www.nadaindia.org/upload_file/document/1493564575.pdf (accessed 5 December 2018)

8 Richa R. Mulchandani, "Doping and Sports in India" in Lovely Dasgupta and Shameek Sen (eds.), Sports Law in India-policy, Regulation and Commercialisation (Sage, 2018)

that are built in the sports institutions of developing countries. As a case in point, one can re-visit the struggles faced by India's star gymnast Dipa Karmakar. Her road to the 2016 Rio Summer Olympics was littered with obstacles. One of her biggest challenges was the lack of an adequate training facility. She trained to learn the Produnova vault with the help of gym mattresses rather than a vault table.[9] Considering that she was training in a facility situated within a state capital speaks volumes about the sports infrastructure in villages and small towns. Added to this is the pressure of winning for the sake of being considered for selection and government grants. PEDs provide a convenient shortcut to winning.[10]

The concerns spelled out in the preceding paragraphs can be further substantiated by reference to the Justice Mudgal committee report. The report was commissioned by the Ministry of Youth Affairs and Sports (MYAS).[11] The terms of reference of the Mudgal Committee, constituted by an Order dated 7th July 2011, was

1   To determine the facts and circumstances leading to large scale recent incidents of alleged doping in the athletics discipline;
2   To examine the reasons for the large scale prevalence of doping, the modus operandi involved, including availability of the prohibited substances in and around training camps/competitions;
3   To enquire into the roles of agencies involved (if any);
4   To suggest remedial measures to improve protocols of dope testing and its integrity and promptness so that such lapses, if any, do not happen in future; and
5   Any other issues.[12]

The document mirrors the problems faced by Indian non-elite athletes by stating that

The athletes, coaches and persons involved with sports in India are still largely unaware of anti-doping programmes. The level of awareness largely varies from complete lack of knowledge to knowing that doping is harmful to the athlete career and health. However only a few have substantial knowledge about anti-doping that is substances and processes banned, the

9 Rimli Bhattacharya, "Dipa Karmakar Faced Unimaginable Odds on Her Journey, But She Never Once Gave Up!" *Women's Web* (2017) www.womensweb.in/2017/12/dipa-karmakar-never-give-up-success-struggle-scars/ (accessed 5 December 2018)
10 *See* Lovely Dasgupta, "Catch Me If You Can! Anti-Doping Policy in India" (2013) www.lawinsport.com/features/item/catch-me-if-you-can-anti-doping-policy-in-india (accessed 5 December 2018)
11 Ministry of Youth Affairs and Sports, *Final Report of the Justice Mudgal Committee Constituted to Probe the Doping Incidents as Per Ministry of Youth Affairs and Sports Order Dated 7th July* (2011) Justice Mudgal (Doping) Probe Committee Report https://docs.google.com/file/d/0By9fMcLYjwJ9X1Zkd3FlYjlrQlk/edit (accessed 5 December 2018)
12 Ibid 2

supplements and food that needs to be avoided, method to take a therapeu-tic exemption, legal avenues available to them in the event of an adverse analytical finding amongst others. NADA needs to consider the economic reality, cultural diversity and the level of education of the Indian athletes, coaches and support personnel when providing education.[13]

The committee recommended that NADA should be free from any governmen-tal influence or that of the National Sports Federation (NSF). Unfortunately, the recommendation, made in 2011, did not seem to have any impact. The current setup of NADA continues to be dominated by government representatives. Con-sequently, the scope of conflict of interest is present and threatens the integrity of NADA. Lack of independence means that decisions are likely to be influenced and customized to suit government interest. Further, there is also the presence of the Indian Olympic Association (IOA) along with other NSFs. This again has the potential of tilting governance-related decisions against the interests of the athletes and other stakeholders. The dominance of powerful groups also means a lack of accountability. This ends up harming the athletes since they continue to be at the mercy of the system. That there are systemic failures in anti-doping implementation measures is also recorded in the Mudgal report. According to the report: "It is seen that there is a general lack of checks and balances in the cur-rent system of sports to ensure that the athletes and their support personnel have understood the concept of anti doping."[14] Hence the committee recommended that NADA should maintain

> [a] record of the people who have attended should be maintained and at the end of the seminar, a certificate/acknowledgement should be given to the athletes/support personnel evidencing their knowledge about anti dop-ing rules and procedures. Alternatively NADA could issue an ID card with a unique number to every attendee to record their attendance and oblige them to sign an acknowledgement that they attended the session/seminar and have understood the basics of the anti doping programme.[15]

The committee also noted lack of personnel and trained support staff for ath-letes. Lack of adequate funding was cited as one of the key factors for the lack of trained personnel. Consequently, the athletes' training was hindered as they lacked access to professional advice on PEDs. A non-elite athlete has to depend on the infrastructure provided by the government through its institutions, like the Sports Authority of India (SAI). Ill-equipped support personnel make the ath-lete vulnerable to being caught in the doping net. The sophisticated anti-doping

13 Ibid 19–20
14 Ibid 22
15 Ibid

measures being developed by WADA means the athletes and their personnel have to be tech-savvy. Unfortunately, for a non-elite developing country athlete this is determined by the kind of government support provided. As the Mudgal report noted:

> the athletes, coaches and support personnel are largely unaware of [ADAMS] and how it works. Therefore each seminar/conference of the NADA should include a practical, simple and effective demonstration of how ADAMS works . . . NADA should seek to provide the information disseminated on ADAMS in the regional languages to the SAI, NIS, Athletes, Coaches and the NSFs. The information should be imparted in simple language avoiding over technical phraseology.[16]

Funding issues continue to be a major problem for non-elite athletes even now. The government support that is given is not adequate to meet the expenses of world-class training.[17] In most cases the athletes fend for themselves. In such a scenario keeping up with high-end WADA compliances is onerous, and athletes are susceptible to making mistakes.[18]

The committee summed up its finding by pointing out the clear lack of accountability amongst the various enforcement agencies. It is the sportsperson who is caught in the crossfire. Each doping incident leads to a blame game, with the concerned authorities passing the buck on to the other. Considering that all the institutions in charge of the anti-doping programme in India are government run, their approach is equally bureaucratic. Hence, no one is willing to acknowledge the inherent flaws within the system. Each decision taken on the issue of WADA Code compliance is based on a reactive approach as opposed to a proactive approach. Though the committee did not address the issue, lack of trained support personnel and anti-doping education means that athletes in India also do not have access to adequate legal advice. This affects their ability to adhere to the obligations under WADA and to understand the implication of the Code provisions. Justice Mudgal rightly concluded that

> The committee finds that the anti-doping programme in India needs an overhaul. The stakeholders in sports are not undertaking adequate positive steps to comply with their obligations under the WADA code. Instead a piece meal system of education is sought to be followed. The stakeholders are constantly involved in shifting the blame to the other stakeholders.

---

16 Ibid 11
17 Rajdeep Puri, "Indian Tennis Woes Spell Dearth of Singles Players" the Quint (New Delhi, 9 November 2018) www.thequint.com/sports/tennis-/problems-in-indian-tennis-lack-of-singles-talent (accessed 5 December 2018)
18 ANI, "Asian Games Bronze Medallist Sells Tea for Living" The Times of India (New Delhi, 7 September 2018) https://timesofindia.indiatimes.com/sports/more-sports/others/asian-games-bronze-medallist-sells-tea-for-living/articleshow/65721615.cms (accessed 5 December 2018)

Each stakeholder needs to understand and implement their duties under the WADA code, instead of following a proactive approach, a reactive approach is being followed where the stakeholders start the process of compliance when a major doping violation occurs.[19]

The reality of a non-elite sporting system in contrast to an elite sports programme thus is documented in the Indian context through the Mudgal report. Houlihan, for instance, points to the perks of elite sports programmes. His research on elite sports in three countries viz. UK, Australia and Canada reveal that there has been an increase in government intervention for the purpose of establishing elite sports programme objectives through the provision of government funds. Additional revenue generation has also been sought through lottery funds. Investments have been made in dedicated world-class facilities suited for elite sportspersons. Additional investment has been made in funding dedicated specialist coaching for the elites. Focus has also been given to elite sports science and sports medicine.[20] No such privileges are found with sports programmes in developing countries. Developing countries have not made large-scale investments in providing world-class facilities. The story of the Indian sports scenario with respect to non-elite athletes holds for other developing countries. For instance, African athletes face similar problems. There, too, athletes are affected by lack of resources and education. Like their Indian counterparts, non-elite African athletes may inadvertently consume PEDs due to their lack of awareness. African athletes thus are victims of their developing country status. Until 2014, Africa had only one laboratory for testing the athletes of fifty-five countries.[21] Consequently, some athletes and support personnel take advantage of the infrastructure crunch, whereas others have no idea that they have used PEDs. Only in August 2018 was a second WADA-accredited laboratory established in Nairobi, Kenya.[22]

The establishment of the Kenyan lab saved Kenya from the prospect of getting sanctioned, given that their leading athletes were under a cloud of suspicion of having doped. In December 2016, WADA conducted an investigation into the issue of doping by Kenyan athletes. WADA partnered with the IAAF Athlete Integrity Unit (AIU) for the investigation and submitted its report on 27 September 2018.[23] The findings of this investigation reaffirms the stated arguments

19 Ministry of Youth Affairs and Sports (n 41)
20 Barrie Houlihan, "Mechanisms of International Influence on Domestic Elite Sport Policy" (2009) 1 (1) *International Journal of Sport Policy and Politics* 51
21 Ntokozo Ayanda Majozi, "Doping, Are There Only a Few Good Apples in the Barrel?" (2014) 2 *African Sports Law and Business Bulletin* 47 www.africansportslawjournal.com/Bulletin_2_2014_Majozi.pdf (accessed 5 December 2018)
22 Reuters, "Sport doping in Kenya 'Uncoordinated, Unsophisticated'-WADA" *The Africa Report* (Nairobi, 28 September 2018) www.theafricareport.com/East-Horn-Africa/sport-doping-in-kenya-uncoordinated-unsophisticated-wada.html (accessed 5 December 2012)
23 WADA, "Doping in Kenya-Stakeholder Project Report" *Intelligence and Investigations Department* www.wada-ama.org/sites/default/files/final_public_report_on_kenya.pdf (accessed 6 December 2018)

on the elite versus non-elite divide. As per the report, Kenyan athletes were involved in "unsophisticated, opportunistic and uncoordinated"[24] doping practices. Clearly the lack of infrastructure and awareness played a major role in such unplanned doping practices. The WADA report confirmed the same by noting that the awareness level of the Kenyan athletes was insufficient.[25] The Kenyan athletes also appeared to be indifferent to the consequences of using PEDs.[26] WADA acknowledged that there was no state-sponsored doping in Kenya, hence it is completely different from an elite, sophisticated doping programme.[27] The report also highlighted the fact that the PEDs used by the Kenyan athletes were primarily over-the-counter medicines. Further, many injected PEDs without any knowledge about the nature of the substances they were consuming.[28] This largely happened in cases where athletes relied on doctors for treatment of their medical conditions. Understandably, with no infrastructural and logistical support it is unfair to expect a non-elite athlete to go about searching for an informed doctor. Consequently, the athletes and their support personnel end up relying on local doctors and chemists for medicines. The local doctors and the chemists are equally unaware of anti-doping issues. They are largely ignorant about the drugs prohibited or permitted by WADA. Accordingly, they are indifferent about what should and should not be given to an athlete.[29] These findings by WADA sum up the scenario that a non-elite athlete is faced with. Unfortunately, the non-elite athletes of developing countries are the voiceless victims of the apathy and elitism that exists in the current anti-doping framework.

ADRV challenges – graveyard for the non-elites

The effect of structural impediments and constraints within non-elite sports programmes is best seen in the cases argued before the CAS. To establish this point, this section will review six cases that have involved Indian athletes and were argued before the CAS. To date, these are the only cases on doping involving Indian athletes that have been arbitrated by the CAS. Hence, they provide a great opportunity to understand the non-elite problem in the current anti-doping system. One of the earliest cases to be argued before the CAS was that of *IAAF v. Akkunji Ashwini*.[30] The concerned athletes tested positive for PEDs. Accordingly, the matter was first referred by NADA to the Anti-Doping

---

24 Ibid 10
25 Ibid
26 Ibid
27 Ibid
28 Ibid 7
29 Ibid 10
30 CAS 2012/A/2763, International Association of Athletics Federations (IAAF) v. Athletics Federation of India (AFI) & Akkunji Ashwini, Priyanka Panwar, Tiana Mary Thomas & Sini Jose, Award of 30 November 2012 (operative part of 17 July 2012)

Disciplinary Panel (ADDP). The ADDP sat as the first-instance hearing panel and analysed the athletes' defense. The athletes put all the blame on their coach and the SAI for the inadvertent doping. They argued that the consumption of a food supplement was done at the direction of their coach, and that therefore the responsibility of their default would lie with the SAI and the coach appointed by the SAI. The ADDP found them to have committed an ADRV under Article 2.2 of the 2009 WADA Code. Considering that the Code applies the strict liability principle, the presence of PEDs in the sample is enough. Hence, the athletes could not avoid the finding of an ADRV by blaming the SAI and the coach.[31] The ADDP however was lenient on the issue of sanctions. The ADDP went along with the athletes on the issue of their lack of choices. The ADDP empathized with the athletes' statement that in India athletes blindly trust and rely on their coaches. The ADDP gave relief to the athletes under Article 10.5.2 of the WADA 2009 Code.[32]

Thus, the ADDP reasoned that

> the athletes were training at NIS Patiala . . . Mr Iurii Ogorodnik gave them a written food supplement program . . . Mr Iurii Ogorodnik had been appointed by the SAI and was not a coach selected or appointed by the athlete. . . . However, in the context of the circumstances of these athletes it has to be borne in mind that SAI used to provide them with food supplements. The athletes could not be expected to verify such supplements provided to them by the authority responsible for sports in the country. . . . There had never been any complaint against Mr Iurii Ogorodnik and he was a world-renowned coach. . . . It was natural for the athletes to have unflinching faith and confidence in the coach. . . . When Mr Iurii Ogorodnik gave the bottles of Ginseng Kinapi Pill to the athletes they had no occasion to suspect that these could be contaminated . . .
> . . . the athletes have been able to establish how the prohibited substance entered their body and that they bear no significant fault or negligence and

---

31 WADA 2009, Article 2.1 .1[It is each Athlete's personal duty to ensure that no Prohibited Substance enters his or her body. Athletes are responsible for any Prohibited Substance or its Metabolites or Markers found to be present in their Samples. Accordingly, it is not necessary that intent, fault, negligence or knowing Use on the Athlete's part be demonstrated in order to establish an anti-doping violation under Article 2.1.]

32 WADA 2009, Article 10.5.2 [No Significant Fault or Negligence If an Athlete or other Person establishes in an individual case that he or she bears No Significant Fault or Negligence, then the otherwise applicable period of Ineligibility may be reduced, but the reduced period of Ineligibility may not be less than one-half of the period of Ineligibility otherwise applicable. If the otherwise applicable period of Ineligibility is a lifetime, the reduced period under this Article may be no less than eight (8) years. When a Prohibited Substance or its Markers or Metabolites is detected in an Athlete's Sample in violation of Article 2.1 (Presence of a Prohibited Substance or its Metabolites or Markers), the Athlete must also establish how the Prohibited Substance entered his or her system in order to have the period of Ineligibility reduced.]

are entitled a reduction in the period of ineligibility under article 10.5.2 of
the rules.

Under article 10.2 read with 10.5.2 ineligibility of one (1) year is imposed
on the athletes . . . for the violation of article 2.1 of Anti-Doping Rules,
NADA. The period of ineligibility shall commence from the date of this
order.

The above quoted reasoning of the ADDP coopts the unique circumstances
of an Indian athlete within the anti-doping narrative. In the Indian context a
coach is treated as a father figure. That explains the institution of an award by
the Indian government to recognize coaches. The award has been named after
one of the most inspiring teachers in Hindu mythology: Dronacharya is the royal
teacher and an important character in the epic Mahabharata. The award is given
to coaches

who have successfully trained sportspersons or teams and enabled them to
achieve outstanding results in International competitions. Dronacharya
Awards are given in two categories (i) Regular Category (ii) Lifetime Category. The Awardees are given a statuette of Guru Dronacharya, a certificate,
ceremonial dress and a cash prize of Rs. 5.00 lakh.[33]

This understanding of the relationship between an athlete and coach explains
the blind trust in the coach. It also indicates a lack of choices and awareness as
far as Indian athletes are concerned because they are under the direct control
and supervision of the SAI. The SAI is under the aegis of the Indian government
through the Ministry of Youth Affairs and Sports. Its governing body is dominated by the representatives of the government of India.[34] For a non-elite athlete,
who feels lucky to get the opportunity to train within SAI's establishment, the
thought of questioning training-related schedules rarely arises. In such a scenario,
the reliance on the coach and the taking of the food supplements was part of
the normal routine. Unlike a developed country elite star athlete, a non-elite
athlete is burdened by circumstances. For the non-elite athletes, coaches are the
key person who can help them attain all of their goals, including team selection,
government grants, stipends and jobs.

The athletes challenged the imposition of the one-year ban and WADA challenged the application of the rule of No-Significant Fault/No-Significant Negligence. The appeal was filed before the Anti-Doping Appeal Panel (ADAP).
The ADAP held that there had been no fault or negligence on the part of the

33 Ministry of Youth Affairs and Sports, "Dronacharya Award" *Government of India* https://yas.nic.in/
dronacharya-award (accessed 5 December 2018)
34 Sports Authority of India, "Governing Body Composition" *Ministry of Youth Affairs and Sports, Government of India* http://sportsauthorityofindia.nic.in/showfile.asp?link_temp_id=5475 (accessed
5 December 2018)

athletes. The ADAP also gave an *in arguendo* by holding that the athletes were not significantly at fault or negligent. The ADAP first evaluated the appeal based on Article 10.5.1 of the 2009 WADA Code.[35] The ADAP noted that

> Since Ginseng had been provided to them by AFI/SAI since years, the Athletes, in good faith, accepted the Ginseng Kianpi Pill as the part of food schedule as being done by them earlier. The Athletes had absolutely no reason to believe that ginseng provided to them would be contaminated or could reasonably be expected to be contaminated because ginseng being a food supplement has regularly been administered and provided by AFI from time to time. Therefore, the Ginseng Kianpi Pill consumed by the Athletes was presumed to be safe, acceptable and permitted and it was not necessary to warrant an investigation about the safety and purity of Ginseng Kianpi Pill.[36]

The ADAP went on to state that

> It is a fallacious argument to suggest that the Athletes were negligent as this Panel is of the view that it was not necessary on the part of the Athletes to enquire about the source or assurances of medical professional regarding purity of the Ginseng Kianpi Pill. It is only when the Athlete suspects or has reason to believe that the supplement might contain a prohibited substance would it be mandatory for them to take steps in terms of the Rules to exercise upmost caution.[37]

According to the ADAP,

> The Athletes in the facts and circumstances were not required to do any comprehensive enquiry and it would be stretching the rules to the limit if it were to hold that every time Ginseng is consumed it was to be tested, this is not the case of WADA. The present case is not a typical case of Doping, it cannot be expected Athletes who has taken Ginseng till the test provided positive were bound to get a test done on each occasion when supplement

---

35 WADA Code 2009, Article 10.5.1 [No Fault or Negligence If an Athlete establishes in an individual case that he or she bears No Fault or Negligence, the otherwise applicable period of Ineligibility shall be eliminated. When a Prohibited Substance or its Markers or Metabolites is detected in an Athlete's Sample in violation of Article 2.1 (Presence of Prohibited Substance), the Athlete must also establish how the Prohibited Substance entered his or her system in order to have the period of Ineligibility eliminated. In the event this Article is applied and the period of Ineligibility otherwise applicable is eliminated, the anti-doping rule violation shall not be considered a violation for the limited purpose of determining the period of Ineligibility for multiple violations under Article 10.7.]
36 CAS 2012/A/2763 (n 30) para 2.21
37 Ibid

was provided by SAI/AFI. It is in fact the duty of the SAI/AFI to have done the exercise if they know or suspected that the coach would give the contaminated supplement.[38]

The last line of the quoted paragraph is significant for it shifts the onus of protecting the athlete onto the Athlete Federation of India (AFI) and the SAI. As mentioned earlier, in the Indian context non-elite athletes are not treated as independent entities free to make their own decisions. On the contrary, the authorities viz. SAI and AFI are regarded as *parens patriae* of the athletes. Hence the liability is vicarious and not personal on the part of the athletes.

Continuing with this line of thought the ADAP held that

> There is no reason for the Panel to assume that every time a supplement/ ginseng is given by AFI/SAI in a routine manner it has to be tested. It is only after the testing of Ginseng Kianpi Pill it was discovered that it was contaminated. Therefore it follows that the Athletes were not at fault or negligent at any stage. However had the test results of the supplements tested by NDTL revealed the source of the prohibited substance in the sample of the athletes was something other than Ginseng Kianpi Pill, the case would have certainly taken a different complexion. The facts of the case are so glaring that to hold that the Athletes are guilty of not exercising upmost caution and care would be doing injustice to the Athletes. Further the Panel cannot lose sight of the fact that the Athletes made no attempt to gain any unfair advantage over other athletes or to enhance their performance.
>
> The Panel in light of the aforesaid discussion has arrived at the conclusion that the Athletes could not have reasonably known or suspected in the facts and circumstances of the present case that Ginseng Kianpi Pill would be contaminated.[39]

For the ADAP the circumstances cited above thus made the cases rarest of rare and thus exceptional. Hence, the ADAP refused to rely on any of the CAS jurisprudence on the issue of doping. The ADAP then goes on to reason *in arguendo* that

> even if the Panel concludes that the Athletes committed some fault the Panel considers that a degree of fault or negligence that they exhibited was so negligible as almost to amount to No Fault or Negligence. In the typical facts and circumstances of the present case the Athletes cannot be said to have deviated from their expected standard of behaviour. The Panel is of the view that it is in the category of these exceptional cases where the extremely

38 Ibid
39 Ibid

strict interpretation of the Rules will produce a result that is neither just nor proportionate in that the totality of the facts and circumstances of the present case and the conditions prevailing in India.[40]

Thus, the ADAP approach gives an alternative viewpoint to the prevailing approach. The ADAP took into account the totality of the circumstances, including the socio-cultural context. This allowed the ADAP to empathize with athletes and understand their viewpoint. The approach of the ADAP holds the authorities in charge of implementing the anti-doping programme responsible. This shifting of the focus from the governed to the governing is a refreshing change that is missing from the current anti-doping discourse.

The ADAP further reduced the period of the athletes' sanction by backdating the starting period to the date of the sample collection. Expectedly, the decision of the ADAP to further reduce the athletes' sanction did not go without challenge. As soon as the IAAF was notified of the ADAP decision it filed an appeal before the CAS. The IAAF pleaded for the imposition of the sanction as mandated under Article 10.2 of the 2009 WADA Code viz. two years.[41] The IAAF argued that India had a serious doping problem and hence the athletes blaming others for their misfortune was incredible.[42] Because the ADRV had been established the athletes had no onus to explain how the PEDs entered their system. Their explanation based on consumption of a food supplement did not appear plausible on the balance of probability. The IAAF buttressed its argument on the basis of the expert testimony as given on behalf of WADA, which declared the brand of Kianpi Pills alleged to be the source had no traces of PEDs. The IAAF alleged that the coach had devised a sophisticated doping programme that involved the ingestion of steroids, since the same had been found in the athletes' samples. The IAAF stated it was not a case of inadvertent doping through a contaminated food supplement. On the issue of elimination of the sanction, the IAAF's position was that even if the Kianpi Pills could be proven to be the source, it still did not merit application of No Significant Fault/Negligence. For the IAAF, there must be exceptional circumstances to convince the panel that the criteria of Article 10.5.2 have been met. The IAAF's ADR were reiterations of the 2009 WADA Code, hence the standard of evaluation had to be the same.

---

40 Ibid
41 WADA Code, 2009, Article 10.2 [The period of Ineligibility imposed for a violation of Article 2.1 (Presence of Prohibited Substance or its Metabolites or Markers), Article 2.2 (Use or Attempted Use of Prohibited Substance or Prohibited Method) or Article 2.6 (Possession of Prohibited Substances and Prohibited Methods) shall be as follows, unless the conditions for eliminating or reducing the period of Ineligibility, as provided in Articles 10.4 and 10.5, or the conditions for increasing the period of Ineligibility, as provided in Articles 10.6, are met: First violation: Two (2) years Ineligibility]
42 CAS 2012/A/2763(n 30) para 5.2

The IAAF further argued that ingestion of contaminated food supplements did not ordinarily amount to exceptional circumstances. It further argued that the conduct of the athletes was not above board because the athletes had spent thousands of rupees to buy supplements from local chemists. As per the IAAF, the athletes never used the supplements as provided by Netaji Subhas National Institute of Sports Patiala (NIS). The most interesting part of the /IAAF's argument was where it pleaded that

> [t]he Athletes were well educated and were all in paid employment with different Government services in India: Ashwini with a national bank, Jose and Panwar with the Indian Railways and Thomas with the Oil and Natural Gas Corporation (Oil India Limited). Further they had travelled internationally and had earned substantial sums from both the Indian Government and sponsors. They had also admitted to having access to the Internet.[43]

This argument de-contextualizes the facts from the socio-cultural setting. The IAAF therefore demonstrated a level of ignorance as well as a lack of understanding of the non-elite athletes' circumstances. As noted earlier, it's precisely because they are doing government jobs that they were not in a position to question the coach appointed by the very same government. Further, the IAAF ignored the fact that appointment to the government organization is based not on educational qualifications but on sports performance. The IAAF's presumption that the athletes are empowered and elite individuals is a far cry from the reality. And access to the internet really does not help when one is entirely subservient to the system.

The IAAF used this incorrect presumption to prove that the athletes were guilty of Significant Fault and Negligence. It substantiated its argument by pointing out that

a   they failed to heed the numerous warnings about supplements;
b   they failed to seek advice from a specialist doctor before taking the supplements;
c   they failed to conduct a basic review of the packaging of the supplements;
d   they failed to conduct any basic internet search about the supplements;
e   they failed to make enquiry of the manufacture or arrange for the supplement to be tested before using them;
f   they failed to exercise due care in not taking other supplements; and
g   the fact of the matter is that the Athletes took no steps at all.[44]

43 Ibid (n 40) para 5.16
44 Ibid para 5.18

The IAAF dismissed the ADAP's reasoning as *"legal abracadabra"* and was dismissive of its approach, including the rationale to back date the sanction. Understandably, the athletes repeated their defense as given to the ADDP and the ADAP. The athletes' arguments thus did add anything new to the existing information that the doping was inadvertent. Further, the athletes did not rely on scientific literature or expert witnesses to explain the nature of the supplement they consumed. No argument was put forth based on data as to the possibility of the contamination of the Kianpi Pills. There were no independent lab reports or tests that the athletes relied upon to substantiate their argument of the contamination of the Kianpi Pills. In short, if one contrasts the arguments as given by an elite developed country athlete with the current case, it is a revelation. It's a revelation of the extent to which a non-elite developing country athlete is vulnerable in the absence of adequate support. In the absence of a solid counterargument based on expert witnesses, the athletes were sitting ducks for the IAAF. They had literally nothing to counter the IAAF on its two most important points viz. burden of proof and elimination/reduction of sanction. Thus, the poverty is not only at the stage of training but also at the stage of litigation. The sophistication with which arbitral proceedings before the CAS are conducted in matters of high-profile athletes is simply missing in the current case.

The athletes ended up arguing that they *"had no knowledge of computers. They had only completed their schooling and the Athletes did not have access to an internet facility at the NIS and they were not allowed to go out of the camp at Patiala."*[45] Another argument they gave was that

> [t]he Athletes were under the impression that the supplements, including the Kianpi Pills, in particular Ginseng were supplied by the AFI via their Coach. Therefore they would not expect to be given something they should not take. It cannot be expected that the Athletes would disbelieve the Government and/or federation. Further, had they failed to follow the Coach's instructions then they would have been kicked off the team.[46]

This argument lacks scientific merit, but it reflects the realities of the system that the non-elite athletes are in. The lack of independent decision making is reflected in the athletes' arguments by the athletes. Another inane argument they make is that "[t]he CAS jurisprudence that the Appellant has submitted does not apply to the facts of this case. There has not been any case involving supplements provided by the athlete's Government."[47] And the best is, "The Athletes did not cheat to win their gold medals in the commonwealth and Asian Games, so why should they cheat now?"[48] These sorts of arguments are not based

45 Ibid (n 30) para 5.28
46 Ibid para 5.38
47 Ibid para 5.40
48 Ibid para 5.42

on legal reasoning or scientific data. Hence, the athletes were bound to fail the WADA test.

For the CAS Panel, it was an easy case. In so far as the discharge of burden of proof of the athletes was concerned, the Panel was convinced that the Kianpi Pills were the source of AAF. The CAS arrived at this conclusion because the IAAF could not prove direct ingestion of steroids. Further, it was on record and undisputed by the IAAF that the athletes were taking a variety of supplements purchased from outside the NIS, and hence the possibility existed of inadvertent doping. The coach also had provided a written statement that he supplied the athletes the pills, purchased from outside. Finally, the test report from the WADA-accredited laboratory at New Delhi also confirmed the presence of steroids in the Kianpi Pills consumed by the athletes. This led the Panel to state that, on the balance of probability, the athletes had discharged their burden of proof. However the tide turned against the athletes on the second issue of elimination/reduction of sanction. Since the arguments on this point were primarily about shifting the onus on AFI/SAI and the coach, clearly the CAS would not be convinced. Accordingly, the CAS reiterated the most important rule of anti-doping viz. "it is each Athletes personal duty to ensure that no prohibited substance enters his body. Athletes are responsible for any prohibited substance or its metabolites or markers found to be present in their samples."[49] Thereafter, the reasoning was on expected lines. The CAS declared that "Athletes cannot shift their responsibility on to third parties simply by claiming that they were acting under instruction or that they were doing what they were told."[50]

The CAS Panel rejected the athletes' argument that they were not warned and that they had no means to know or even determine what they were consuming. The CAS went by the statements of Indian officials in charge of the anti-doping programme, who understandably claimed that they did all as per their compliance requirement. In other words, the fault was solely on the athletes, who, as the CAS said, ignored all the education and awareness they received from the Indian government agency on food supplements. The CAS, too, had de-contextualized the debate and ignored the non-elite context by stating that

> as international athletes competing at the level that the Athletes competed, it is somewhat unbelievable that the Athletes can submit that they were not aware of the risk of taking supplements and had received no education or warnings at all. Whilst the level of anti-doping education in India does not appear to be at a satisfactory level and perhaps not as developed as in many other parts of the World, there does appear to be some basic education and/or warnings given at the NIS.[51]

49 Ibid para 9.19
50 Ibid para 9.22
51 Ibid para 9.23

Amongst all this, the CAS also was forced to note the obvious lack of effort in conducting education programmes by NADA, NIS, SAI and others. However, this acknowledgement of the institutional faults did not save the day for the athletes as the strict liability norm rules and the personal liability of the athlete superseded all intervening factors.

The CAS put the onus on the athletes to seek expert medical advice before consuming the pills. Considering that the in-house doctor admittedly did not have the expertise, this begs the question as to where and how they should seek this advice. Further, the CAS proceeded on the assumption as to the way the in-house doctor would have guided the athletes. This is borne out by the circumstances where the one determining the consumption of the pills was the coach and thus the dominant entity. The CAS thus held that

> the Athletes in this matter did not take any of the reasonable steps expected of them before taking such a supplement and neither did the Coach. Further, the Athletes in this matter had either themselves or had the Coach purchased many other supplements for them to use from the open market. They also consumed a number of supplements and not just simply the one which, on the balance of probabilities, caused the adverse analytical finding.[52]

One of the steps CAS expected from the athletes was that they should have "at the very least asked the Coach from where the supplements had been purchased."[53] This scenario again, given the context, was not necessarily feasible, as noted by the ADAP. Another interesting fact was that CAS acknowledged that

> the Athletes may not be deemed informed athletes due to the complete lack of education that they had been provided the First Respondent and in general in India. However, as explained above, the Sole Arbitrator believes that the Athletes must have been aware of the basic risks of contamination of food supplements.[54]

There appears to be a contradiction here, because if there is no education, how one can expect the athletes to take steps on the basis of the same?

This contradiction is reflected further by the following statement by the CAS that "there were sufficient facilities and personnel available at the NIS training centre which the Athletes were negligent not to use."[55] If this were the case, then there should not have been a lack of education as the personnel available and the facilities available should cater to making the athletes informed. The athletes were imposed with a sanction period of two years since they failed to

52 Ibid para 9.27
53 Ibid para 9.28
54 Ibid para 9.31
55 Ibid para 9.32

discharge the burden of proving No Significant Fault/Negligence. As a measure of tokenism CAS concluded the discussion by giving an advisory to the governing bodies including IAAF to improve the anti-doping awareness programme in India.[56] The other cases involving Indian athletes that came before CAS met the same fate. They all suffered from poorly drafted arguments and a lack of sufficient and sophisticated scientific evidence. The case of IAAF v. *Athletics Federation of India (AFI) & Mandeep Kaur & Jauna Murmu*[57] is in point. The facts are similar to the previous case of Ashwini and Priyanka, as this too dealt with consumption of food supplements. Here too the same coach and the same pill was involved. On the finding of AAF, the matter was referred to ADDP and, like in the previous case, the defense was the same and the reasoning of ADDP was also same. The context of India and the athlete-coach relationship formed the crux of the reasoning. Further the fault of SAI/AFI and the coach was the focus and not that of the athletes. Accordingly, as in the previous case, the athletes were found to have proved No Significant Fault/Negligence. Consequentially the sanction period was reduced to one year. IAAF, expectedly appealed to CAS and pleaded same grounds as in the previous case. The counter of the athletes was also on similar lines as in the previous case. Accordingly, the finding of CAS on all the issues was the same and the sanction of two years was imposed on the athletes, in absence of proof of No Significant Fault/Negligence.[58]

Another case highlighting similar problems of inadequate argument is *World Anti-Doping Agency (WADA) v. Nirupama Devi Laishram.*[59] The athlete tested positive for a specified stimulant prohibited in competition.[60] On the matter being heard by the ADDP, the athlete was given a reprimand without imposing any period of ineligibility. On appeal to the ADAP by NADA, the decision of the ADDP was upheld. On being notified of the same, WADA filed its appeal before the CAS. The locus of WADA was based on the NADA ADR which incorporates the provisions of the WADA Code.[61] NADA ADR Article 13.2.3

56 Ibid para 9.34
57 CAS 2012/A/2732 International Association of Athletics Federations (IAAF) v. Athletics Federation of India (AFI) & Mandeep Kaur & Jauna Murmu, award of 30 November 2012 (operative part of 17 July 2012)
58 Ibid para 9.33
59 CAS 2012/A/2979 World Anti-Doping Agency (WADA) v. Nirupama Devi Laishram & National Anti-Doping Agency of India (NADA), award of 8 November 2013
60 Ibid para 4
61 WADA 2009, Article 13.2.2 and Article 13.2.3 deals with the right to appeal and who can appeal to CAS [13.2.2- Appeals Involving National-level Athletes In cases involving national-level Athletes, as defined by each National Anti-Doping Organization, who do not have a right to appeal under Article 13.2.1, the decision may be appealed to an independent and impartial body in accordance with rules established by the National Anti-Doping Organization. The rules for such appeal shall respect the following principles: • a timely hearing; • a fair, impartial and independent hearing panel; • the right to be represented by counsel at the Person's own expense; and • a timely, written, reasoned decision.] [13.2.3- ... For cases under Article 13.2.2, WADA and the

read with Article 13.2.2 gives WADA the right to appeal to the CAS.[62] The athlete had no argument against the AAF and accepted the finding on the issue of the ADRV without challenge. Hence the only issue was with respect to the period of sanction. In the absence of any proof for reduction/elimination of sanction, the period would be two years for the ADRV as per Article 2.1 of the 2009 WADA Code, as adopted by NADA.[63] To prove her claims for reduction of the sanction, the athlete gave quite flimsy arguments. She claimed that the source of the specified stimulant was VLCC products. Since she was using these products at the time of her positive test, it was thus a case of inadvertent doping. Further, the amount of PED found in her sample was not enough to give her any advantage in performance.

Under the 2009 WADA Code and NADA ADR, Article 10.4 dealt with elimination/reduction of sanction in case of specified substances.[64] Since this case was an ADRV for a specified stimulant, the athlete relied on Article 10.4 in addition to Article 10.5.1.[65] She argued lack of intent to enhance her performance to satisfy the criteria of Article 10.4. Before the CAS Panel the athlete thus had to first prove the source of the specified substance.[66] WADA argued that the athlete had failed to prove she was using VLCC products, since she could not show any receipt of purchase.[67] WADA contended further that even if VLCC was proven to have been used by the athlete at the relevant point in time, it could not be the source of the PED.[68] WADA based its argument on the scientific data which proved that geranium oil, one of the ingredients in VLCC products does not contain the stimulant found in her sample.[69] Importantly, neither VLCC nor NADA's test result revealed the presence of the specified stimulant

---

International Federation shall also have the right to appeal to CAS with respect to the decision of the national-level reviewing body.]

62 NADA Anti-Doping Rules, 2009 (Same as WADA 2009)

63 CAS 2012/A/2979 (n 60) para 30

64 WADA Code 2009, Article 10.4 [Elimination or Reduction of the Period of Ineligibility for Specified Substances under Specific Circumstances Where an Athlete or other Person can establish how a Specified Substance entered his or her body or came into his or her Possession and that such Specified Substance was not intended to enhance the Athlete's sport performance or mask the Use of a performance-enhancing substance, the period of Ineligibility found in Article 10.2 shall be replaced with the following: First violation: At a minimum, a reprimand and no period of Ineligibility from future Events, and at a maximum, two (2) years of Ineligibility. To justify any elimination or reduction, the Athlete or other Person must produce corroborating evidence in addition to his or her word which establishes to the comfortable satisfaction of the hearing panel the absence of an intent to enhance sport performance or mask the Use of a performance-enhancing substance. The Athlete's or other Person's degree of fault shall be the criterion considered in assessing any reduction of the period of Ineligibility.]

65 WADA Code 2009 (n 36)

66 CAS 2012/A/2979 (n 60) para 36

67 Ibid para 37

68 Ibid para 38

69 Ibid para 39

methylhexaneamine.[70] WADA also contended that the amount of methylhexaneamine found in her sample could not be the source of absorption through the skin,[71] and that the amount was sufficient to give her performance advantage.[72] On the whole, the VLCC products did not appear to be the source of the prohibited substance.[73]

The athlete stuck to her argument of VLCC being the source of the prohibited substance.[74] She produced medical literature to support her theory of absorption through the skin.[75] The problem was establishing that VLCC products contained methylhexaneamine. Her argument was accepted before the ADDP, and she was let off with a reprimand and no period of ineligibility as per Article 10.4. On appeal to the ADAP, the decision of the ADDP was upheld, rejecting NADA's contention against cutaneous absorption or absorption through the skin. However it was a completely different scenario before the CAS. On the debate of whether geranium could be the source of methylhexaneamine, WADA's stance appears conflicting. Based on the information on its website at that point in time, it appeared that WADA regarded geranium oil as a potential source of methylhexaneamine.[76] This was in contrast to the stance it took later, as mentioned above. NADA followed the steps of WADA and put up a warning in 2012 that geranium oil could be a source of methylhexaneamine,[77] but NADA did not inform athletes about the potential danger of geranium oil prior to 2012. Hence the athlete here was clearly unaware of the effect of geranium oil and its potential to lead to an AAF. NADA does admit its fault by stating that "the Athlete had no information or clear warning available to her that a geranium based product including that of a beauty product, could result in a prohibited substance entering her body."[78]

NADA's fault thus appears to be a causal factor in the athlete's AAF, as is pointed out in NADA's submission that "the Athlete, therefore, had never been sufficiently warned over the last few years about any substance that may contain methylhexaneamine."[79] Interestingly, WADA's website also reveals that WADA had in 2012 revealed the possibility of methylhexaneamine leading to inadvertent doping.[80] The CAS was thus required to determine whether on the basis of submissions the athlete could receive the benefit of Article 10.4. Considering that the athlete could procure only one piece of medical literature to support her contention of cutaneous absorption, she had a tall order to match. WADA not only procured statements from the VLCC product manufacturer but also had the

70 Ibid para 40–41
71 Ibid para 42
72 Ibid para 43
73 Ibid para 44
74 Ibid para 49
75 Ibid para 51
76 Ibid para 59
77 Ibid para 60
78 Ibid para 61
79 Ibid para 62
80 Ibid para 65

NADA test report. None of these supported the athlete's contention. WADA's most convincing evidence was the statement of Dr Irene Mazzoni, Senior Manager, WADA Science. Her submission was that

> Cutaneous absorption of essential oils including geranium oils is reported to be poor. Therefore, even if the VLCC products did contain methylhexaneamine originating from the geranium oil, cutaneous absorption of methylhexaneamine would be very poor as well. It is therefore extremely unlikely that the normal use of an aesthetic product containing geranium oil would result in a positive test for methylhexaneamine, in particular with such a high urinary concentration.[81]

The CAS did take note of WADA's changing stance on the correlation between geranium oil and methylhexaneamine, and thus was willing to give the benefit of doubt to the athlete on this point.[82] However, CAS rejected the argument of conflict of interest vis-à-vis Dr Mazzoni.

Dr Mazzoni's submission was accepted by the CAS.[83] The athlete's inability to counter the statements that VLCC products did not have methylhexaneamine led the CAS to uphold WADA's plea.[84] The dearth of scientific research to prove her claims again reflects poorly on the help that a non-elite athlete from a developing country gets. One needed an advanced level of scientific research material to debate the issue of cutaneous absorption. Unfortunately, the athlete had none to match the stature or expertise of Dr Mazzonni. The CAS imposed a sanction of two years, subject to deductions. Thus, the CAS took into account the delays caused without her being at fault when determining the start date of her ineligibility period.[85]

Another case which again proves the lack of awareness among non-elite developing country athletes is the case of *World Anti-Doping Agency (WADA) v. Amit*.[86] Here the situation is worse due to the young age of the concerned athlete. The athlete participated in a junior national competition in wrestling. As soon as the competition was over he was selected randomly for dope testing. He refused to sign the notification and ran away from the scene. The next day he voluntarily provided his sample and there was no AAF upon testing. However, his refusal was regarded as an ADRV under WADA Code 2009 Article 2.3[87] The NADA

---

81 Ibid para 113
82 Ibid para 114
83 Ibid para 115
84 Ibid para 116
85 Ibid para 120
86 CAS 2014/A/3869 World Anti-Doping Agency (WADA) v. Amit and National Anti-Doping Agency of India (NADA), award of 23 November 2015
87 WADA Code 2009, Article 2.3 [Refusing or failing without compelling justification to submit to Sample collection after notification as authorized in applicable anti-doping rules, or otherwise evading Sample collection]

ADDP imposed on him an ineligibility period of one year. WADA challenged the same before the ADAP, but the same was dismissed upholding the decision of the ADDP. The ADDP accepted the explanation given by athlete viz. "that someone had informed him that he would fail a doping test as a result of having consumed Red Bull energy drink. He said that it was for this reason that he ran away after being notified of the doping control."[88] WADA accordingly appealed to the CAS against the decision of the ADAP. Here, too, the main issue was the applicability of Article 10.5.1 or Article 10.5.2 since the finding of an ADRV was not challenged. Once again the athlete's lack of awareness and rural background was cited as one of the mitigating factors to establishing the requirements of Article 10.5.2.[89] The CAS had already rejected the applicability of Article 10.5.1 since running away cannot be regarded as no negligence or fault. Understandably, as in the previous cases, the arguments and defenses fell flat. The explanation based on reasons such as the athlete becoming panicked or relying on third-party advice was not good enough and was rejected in accordance with Article 10.5.2. Conjectures could not save the day, and the fact that the sample, when finally given, did not return AAF was again not helpful because it neither proves nor disproves doping. The act was the running away from the scene, and the only explanation was lack of awareness, which as seen earlier would not help. Consequently, the CAS's two-year period of ineligibility was imposed.[90]

World Anti-Doping Agency (WADA) v. Indian National Anti-Doping Agency (NADA) & Mhaskar Meghali[91] is another case involving equally naïve arguments. The athlete tested positive and was found to have committed an ADRV. Her argument was that she was the victim of other players' jealousy.[92] The ADDP reduced her sanction period to one year by applying the rule of No Significant Fault/Negligence.[93] WADA appealed against the ADDP's decision before the CAS, arguing that the period of sanction imposed was erroneous.[94] WADA relied on Article 10.2.1 of the NADA ADR which incorporated the 2015 WADA Code.[95] Thus the period of ineligibility had to be four years as per WADA.[96] To reduce the same, the source of the substance had to be established. This was a requirement for both No Fault/Negligence and No Significant Fault/Negligence. In the absence of proof of the source of the PED, intentional

---

88 CAS 2014/A/3869 (n 87) para 10
89 Ibid para 51
90 Ibid para 60–61
91 CAS 2016/A/4626 World Anti-Doping Agency (WADA) v. Indian National Anti-Doping Agency (NADA) & Mhaskar Meghali, award of 20 September 2016
92 Ibid para 10
93 Ibid para 11
94 Ibid para 25
95 WADA 2015, Article 10.2.1 [The period of Ineligibility shall be four years where: 10.2.1.1 The anti-doping rule violation does not involve a Specified Substance, unless the Athlete or other Person can establish that the anti-doping rule violation was not intentional.]
96 CAS 2014/A/3869 (n 87) para 25

consumption was proven, and thus the four-year period of the sanction.[97] The CAS evaluated the applicability of the definition of intention as given in Article 10.2.3 of the 2015 WADA Code.[98] Thus, the lack of knowledge or lack or inherent risk needs to be proven through balance of probability and an established lack of intention to dope.[99] However in this case the athlete, at the time of hearing before the ADDP, produced a medical prescription to show that she had taken medications on medical advice, essentially trying to prove that the source of the dope was the medication. WADA countered this argument by showing that none of the drugs prescribed contained the PED, methandienone, found in her sample. This nullified the argument of lack of intention.[100] Further, the athlete had not disclosed these medications on her doping control form nor had she sought a TUE. Hence, the source of the substance in her sample was not established.[101]

The ADDP did not require any alternative explanation and presumed based on the prescription itself that the AAF was caused by the medication, and hence there was lack of intention.[102] The ADDP also accepted the argument of jealousy as a proof of lack of intention. Clearly none of these were arguments which could prove a case as per the WADA Code. On the contrary, the whole approach, from the submission of the athlete's arguments to the decision of the ADDP, appeared to be a shoddy affair, which brings forth the fact that non-elite athletes from developing countries continue to remain ill-equipped to deal with anti-doping issues. With increasing stringency in the provisions of the Code, the worst sufferer will be the non-elite athlete. In this case the athlete was imposed the sanction period of four years, as per the 2015 WADA Code, by the CAS.[103]

The last case that will be used to highlight the apathy and the inadequacy of a non-elite athlete vis-à-vis WADA is *WADA v. Narsingh Yadav*.[104] This case was decided by the Ad Hoc Division of CAS for the 2016 Rio Summer Olympics. There was infighting between the athlete, Narsingh Yadav, and his competitor and rival Sushil Kumar. On 5 June 2016, Chandan, a partner of Yadav, alleged that another wrestler from Kumar's camp had contaminated food prepared for Yadav. Yadav was unaware of the act of contamination. Sometime later in the month of June 2016 Yadav alleged that his energy drink had been

97 Ibid para 27–28
98 WADA Code 2015, Article 10.2.3 [the term "intentional" is meant to identify those Athletes who cheat. The term, therefore, requires that the Athlete or other Person engaged in conduct which he or she knew constituted an anti-doping rule violation or knew that there was a significant risk that the conduct might constitute or result in an anti-doping rule violation and manifestly disregarded that risk.]
99 CAS 2014/A/3869 (n 87) para 45
100 Ibid para 46–47
101 Ibid para 47
102 Ibid para 50
103 Ibid para 51
104 CAS OG 16/25 WADA v Narsingh Yadav and NADA

contaminated by a wrestler from Kumar's camp. Soon after this declaration, Yadav underwent an out-of-competition test. His roommate and training partner was also tested. In July, another out-of-competition sample was collected from Yadav. On 15 July both Yadav and his roommate and training partner tested positive for AAF.

During the course of the hearing before the NADA ADDP, Yadav pleaded sabotage and contamination of his drink by Kumar's camp. The list of nutritional and food supplements that the athlete provided to the NADA did not reveal the presence of any PED. Hence, the ADDP was keen to accept the argument of sabotage and applied No Fault/Negligence. The ADDP accordingly applied Article 10.4 of the 2015 WADA Code.[105] WADA appealed before the CAS Ad Hoc Division against the ADDP, since the athlete had proceeded to participate in the Rio Olympics. WADA argued that his participation was the outcome of the ADDP decision, and hence the dispute was in connection with the Olympic Games. This meant that the CAS Ad Hoc Division thus had jurisdiction.[106] The CAS accepted this submission and proceeded to hear and decide the matter. WADA as usual relied on scientific evidence to argue that the athlete had failed to prove the source of the PED, methandienone, that had been found in the athlete's sample.[107] Hence, the act was intentional and needed to be sanctioned with four years of ineligibility, as per the 2015 WADA Code.[108] WADA relied on the expert evidence of Dr Christiane Ayotte to disprove the theory of sabotage and to prove the theory of intentional doping.[109] The only argument the athlete relied upon was sabotage. The athlete tried to prove the same by citing the fact that a police complaint had been filed for attempted sabotage. However, the athlete's argument lacked any scientific evidence or expert witness to counter WADA.[110]

As in the previous cases, the CAS Panel had no option but to conclude that "the Athlete has failed to satisfy his burden of proof,"[111] with the most likely explanation being that the athlete had consumed the PED intentionally. A four-year sanction was imposed on the athlete. These cases involving Indian athletes mirror the impediments due not only to lack of awareness but also to the poor quality of evidentiary material produced before the CAS Panels. Added to this is the pro-elite assumptions that exist regarding the extent of accessibility and knowledge and other privileges that an international athlete is presumed to have. The personal circumstances and context are ignored, and thus the non-elite

---

105 WADA Code 2015, Article 10.4 [Elimination of the Period of Ineligibility where there is No Fault or Negligence If an Athlete or other Person establishes in an individual case that he or she bears No Fault or Negligence, then the otherwise applicable period of Ineligibility shall be eliminated.]
106 CAS OG 16/25 (n 105) para 5.6
107 Ibid para 7.3
108 Ibid para 7.6
109 Ibid para 7.13
110 Ibid para 7.7–7.11
111 Ibid para 7.27

athlete is put in a no-win situation. In contrast, the personal situation of an elite athlete is poles apart. Hence, when such an athlete bases their arguments on personal flaws the standard of evaluation ought to be more stringent. For instance, when Maria Sharapova was caught using a PED, she expressed ignorance of the fact that "the active ingredient of Mildronate, a medication which she had regularly been using for over 10 years, had been added to the Prohibited List from 1 January 2016 and she did not intentionally contravene the anti-doping rules in using Mildronate at the Australian Open."[112] This argument ideally cannot be accepted precisely because Sharapova, before testing positive for AAF, was the richest female athlete in the world.[113] Importantly, this argument is no different from the argument that Ashwini and others gave about their lack of knowledge. The circumstances of the non-elite Indian athlete sharply contrasts with the privileges Sharapova has. She has access to the best personnel as her support staff. Hence, complying with the requirements of WADA, such as being constantly updated about the Prohibited List, should have been easy.

That Sharapova and her support staff have always been careful about complying with WADA was evidenced by the proceedings before the International Tennis Federation (ITF) Tribunal (hereinafter the Tribunal). The evidence shows that Sharapova has always been WADA Code compliant. For instance, when medications were recommended for treating a viral condition, Sharapova insisted that

> any substances . . . recommended must comply with the WADA Code. So . . . the substances . . . recommended [were] reviewed by the Director of the WADA accredited laboratory at the Moscow anti-doping centre. On 11 January 2006 the centre reported that the 18 pharmaceutical preparations listed, including Mildronate, did not contain substances included on the 2006 Prohibited List.[114]

This level of awareness needs to be provided to the non-elite developing country athlete. Unfortunately, they are not provided with the wherewithal to have access to this level of awareness. If after such precautions even Sharapova can fall afoul of the ever-changing WADA Code, one has no option but to empathize with the situation of a non-elite developing country athlete. Unfortunately, when applying the principle of No Significant Fault/Negligence, the CAS Panel does not perceive this inherent difficulty. On the contrary, they appear to be more sympathetic towards the elite star athlete. In the case of Sharapova, for instance, the CAS, while assessing her appeal against the ITF ban, applied the

---

112 The International Tennis Federation v. Maria Sharapova para 6

113 "Why Everyone in Tennis Hates Maria Sharapova" *News.com.au* (New South Wales, 30 March 2016) www.news.com.au/sport/tennis/why-everyone-in-tennis-hates-maria-sharapova/news-(story/86b48228494b5392ee0adc0183cf7523 (accessed 5 November 2018)

114 Maria Sharapova (n 113) para 23

principle of No Significant Fault/Negligence under Article 10.5.2 of the 2015 WADA Code.[115] And one of the reasons given for reducing Sharapova's sanction based on No Significant Fault/Negligence was that

> no specific warning had been issued by the relevant organizations (WADA, ITF or WTA) as to the change in the status of Meldonium (the ingredient of Mildronate). In that respect, the Panel notes that anti-doping organizations should have to take reasonable steps to provide notice to athletes of significant changes to the Prohibited List, such as the addition of a substance, including its brand names.[116]

This lack of information and awareness was the argument given in the cases discussed earlier, but the CAS did not regard that as a ground to be considered for the applicability of No Significant Fault/Negligence. The point being that the WADA Code implementation needs to co-opt the non-elite perspective. There needs to be an understanding of the non-elite athlete's problem. There needs to be a revisiting of the WADA Code provisions to incorporate the non-elite discourse. The missing link in the current anti-doping discourse is the non-elite perspective. It needs to be included while discussing the anti-doping issues. The Richard Gasquet case[117] is an eye-opener as to the extent to which a non-elite athlete lacks in resources. Gasquet was accused of using cocaine in competition, and he took the defense of No Fault and Negligence. Gasquet convinced the CAS to rule out deliberate ingestion of cocaine through expert witnesses.[118] He used expert witnesses to prove that the amount of cocaine found in his sample was the result of contamination.[119] He had an expert witness agree to the point that "contamination with cocaine through kissing is, from a medical point of view, a possibility in the present case."[120] Having proven such an extraordinary argument, upholding the plea of No Fault/Negligence was just a formality.

115 WADA Code 2015, Article 10.5.2 [If an Athlete or other Person establishes in an individual case where Article 10.5.1 is not applicable, that he or she bears No Significant Fault or Negligence, then, subject to further reduction or elimination as provided in Article 10.6, the otherwise applicable period of Ineligibility may be reduced based on the Athlete or other Person's degree of Fault, but the reduced period of Ineligibility may not be less than one-half of the period of Ineligibility otherwise applicable. If the otherwise applicable period of Ineligibility is a lifetime, the reduced period under this Article may be no less than eight years.]

116 CAS 2016/A/4643 Maria Sharapova v. International Tennis Federation (ITF), award of 30 September 2016, para 92

117 Arbitration CAS 2009/A/1926 International Tennis Federation (ITF) v. Richard Gasquet & CAS 2009/A/1930 World Anti-Doping Agency (WADA) v. ITF & Richard Gasquet, award of 17 December 2009

118 Ibid para 33

119 Ibid para 42

120 Ibid para 46

For the CAS, Gasquet's act of kissing Pamela, the girl to who he was attracted to in the night club, could not be regarded as faulty or negligent because "the Player could not have been aware of the consequences that kissing Pamela could have on him. It was simply impossible for the Player, even when exercising the utmost caution, to know that in kissing Pamela, he could be contaminated with cocaine."[121] The CAS further noted that

> it was impossible for the Player to know, still exercising the utmost caution, that when indeed kissing Pamela, she might inadvertently administer cocaine to him. As the Player did not know Pamela's cocaine history and did not see her, during the entire evening, taking cocaine or appearing to be under its influence, how could he imagine that she had been consuming cocaine? And even more, how should he have been in a position to know that, even assuming that he knew that she had been consuming cocaine, that it was medically possible to be contaminated with cocaine by kissing someone who had ingested cocaine beforehand?[122]

Thus, sophistication is needed to prove any argument before CAS. And sophistication can only come through the availability of resources or else it will be a situation where the non-elite will end up dead and defeated in the graveyard trying to negotiate the WADA Code.

Conclusion

On 27 February 2018 the UK Parliament published a report on doping in sport.[123] Apart from everything else, what the report revealed was the abuse of TUEs for performance enhancement. The sport in respect of which this finding was published was British Cycling. The star performer whose TUE was under scrutiny was Sir Bradley Wiggins.[124] The report concluded that TUEs were being abused for gaining performance enhancement. These findings exemplify the advantages that the elite take or are in a position to take in the current anti-doping regime. However, as one saw in the case of developing countries like Kenya and India, the non-elite athletes are not anywhere near abusing the system. They don't even have the means to abuse, and that is precisely the reason they get caught so easily. The divide between the elite and the non-elite

121 Ibid para 53
122 Ibid
123 House of Commons Digital, Culture, Media and Sport Committee, *Combatting Doping in Sport-fourth Report of Session 2017–19* (27 February 2018) https://publications.parliament.uk/pa/cm201719/cmselect/cmcumeds/366/366.pdf (accessed 6 December 2018)
124 Martha Kelner, "Bradley Wiggins and Team Sky Accused in Damning Drugs Report" *The Guardian* (London, 5 March 2018) www.theguardian.com/sport/2018/mar/05/bradley-wiggins-and-team-sky-accused-drugs-in-damning-reportn (accessed 6 December 2018)

cannot be abridged with system changes. On the contrary, every new stringency in the WADA Code affects the rights of the non-elite to be treated fairly. This affects their ability to use the existing processes to prove their innocence. The scrutiny of the CAS decisions in this chapter revealed how poorly the arguments are made. There is no support system to help athletes once they are caught, and there is no system to instill accountability amongst anti-doping agencies.

Bibliography

ANI, "Asian Games Bronze Medallist Sells Tea for Living" *The Times of India* (New Delhi, 7 September 2018) https://timesofindia.indiatimes.com/sports/more-sports/others/asian-games-bronze-medallist-sells-tea-for-living/articleshow/65721615.cms (accessed 5 December 2018)

Arbitration CAS 2009/A/1926 International Tennis Federation (ITF) v. Richard Gasquet & CAS 2009/A/1930 World Anti-Doping Agency (WADA) v. ITF & Richard Gasquet, award of 17 December 2009

Australian Government, Australian Anti-Doping Authority https://elearning.asada.gov.au/ (accessed 5 December 2018)

Bhattacharya, Rimli, "Dipa Karmakar Faced Unimaginable Odds on Her Journey, But She Never Once Gave Up!" *Women's Web* (2017) www.womensweb.in/2017/12/dipa-karmakar-never-give-up-success-struggle-scars/ (accessed 5 December 2018)

CAS 2012/A/2732, International Association of Athletics Federations (IAAF) v. Athletics Federation of India (AFI) & Mandeep Kaur & Jauna Murmu, award of 30 November 2012 (operative part of 17 July 2012)

CAS 2012/A/2763, International Association of Athletics Federations (IAAF) v. Athletics Federation of India (AFI) & Akkunji Ashwini, Priyanka Panwar, Tiana Mary Thomas & Sini Jose, award of 30 November 2012 (operative part of 17 July 2012)

CAS 2012/A/2979, World Anti-Doping Agency (WADA) v. Nirupama Devi Laishram & National Anti-Doping Agency of India (NADA), award of 8 November 2013

CAS 2014/A/3869, World Anti-Doping Agency (WADA) v. Amit and National Anti-Doping Agency of India (NADA), award of 23 November 2015

CAS 2016/A/4626, World Anti-Doping Agency (WADA) v. Indian National Anti-Doping Agency (NADA) & Mhaskar Meghali, award of 20 September 2016

CAS 2016/A/4643, Maria Sharapova v. International Tennis Federation (ITF), award of 30 September 2016, para 92

CAS OG 16/25, WADA v Narsingh Yadav and NADA

Dasgupta, Lovely, "Catch Me If You Can! Anti-Doping Policy in India" www.lawinsport.com/features/item/catch-me-if-you-can-anti-doping-policy-in-india (accessed 5 December 2018)

Dictionary.com www.dictionary.com/browse/developing-country (accessed 5 December 2018)

Houlihan, Barrie, "Mechanisms of International Influence on Domestic Elite Sport Policy" (2009) 1 (1) *International Journal of Sport Policy and Politics* 51

House of Commons Digital, Culture, Media and Sport Committee, *Combatting Doping in Sport-fourth Report of Session 2017–19* (27 February 2018) https://publications.parliament.uk/pa/cm201719/cmselect/cmcumeds/366/366.pdf (accessed 6 December 2018)

The International Tennis Federation v. Maria Sharapova

Kelner, Martha, "Bradley Wiggins and Team Sky Accused in Damning Drugs Report" *The Guardian* (London, 5 March 2018) www.theguardian.com/sport/2018/mar/05/bradley-wiggins-and-team-sky-accused-drugs-in-damning-reportn (accessed 6 December 2018)

Ministry of Youth Affairs and Sports, "Dronacharya Award" *Government of India* https://yas.nic.in/dronacharya-award (accessed 5 December 2018)

Ministry of Youth Affairs and Sports, *Final Report of the Justice Mudgal Committee Constituted to Probe the Doping Incidents as Per Ministry of Youth Affairs and Sports Order Dated 7th July 2011* (2011) Justice Mudgal (Doping) Probe Committee Report https://docs.google.com/file/d/0By9fMcLYjwJ9X1Zkd3FlYjlrQlk/edit (accessed 5 December 2018)

Mulchandani, Richa R., "Doping and Sports in India" in Lovely Dasgupta and Shameek Sen (eds.), *Sports Law in India-policy, Regulation and Commercialisation* (Sage, 2018)

NADA, "Anti-Doping Awareness Program Conducted by NADA" (April 2018 to June 2018) www.nadaindia.org/upload_file/document/1532087561.pdf (accessed 5 December 2018)

NADA, "Publications" www.nadaindia.org/upload_file/document/1493564575.pdf (accessed 5 December 2018)

NADA, "Publications" www.nadaindia.org/en/publication-books (accessed 6 December 2018)

Ntokozo, Ayanda Majozi, "Doping, Are There Only a Few Good Apples in the Barrel?" (2014) 2 *African Sports Law and Business Bulletin* 47

Prabhu, Dinesh, "Sports Jobs 2019 – Sports Quota Recruitment (16 Govt Vacancies) *IndGovtJobs* (2018) www.indgovtjobs.in/2014/07/Sports-Quota-Recruitment.html (accessed 5 December 2018)

Puri, Rajdeep, "Indian Tennis Woes Spell Dearth of Singles Players" *The Quint* (New Delhi, 9 November 2018) www.thequint.com/sports/tennis-/problems-in-indian-tennis-lack-of-singles-talent (accessed 5 December 2018)

Reuters, "Sport Doping in Kenya 'Uncoordinated, Unsophisticated'-WADA" The Africa Report (Nairobi, 28 September 2018) www.theafricareport.com/East-Horn-Africa/sport-doping-in-kenya-uncoordinated-unsophisticated-wada.html (accessed 5 December 2012)

Sports Authority of India, "Governing Body Composition" *Ministry of Youth Affairs and Sports, Government of India* http://sportsauthorityofindia.nic.in/showfile.asp?link_temp_id=5475 (accessed 5 December 2018)

WADA 2009

WADA Code 2015

WADA, "Doping in Kenya-stakeholder Project Report" *Intelligence and Investigations Department* www.wada-ama.org/sites/default/files/final_public_report_on_kenya.pdf (accessed 6 December 2018)

"Why Everyone in Tennis Hates Maria Sharapova" *News.com.au* (New South Wales, 30 March 2016)

Chapter 5

Changing the anti-doping narrative

Time to incorporate the subaltern discourse

Introduction

Having forcefully argued in the previous chapter for the need to change the perspective and the contours of the debate, this chapter provides ideas that might bring about much-needed reform. The disclaimer is that the ideas are not new or novel. However, in the context of all that has happened since the Russian doping scandal, one has to look into the issues of transparency and accountability. Reform has to be introduced at three levels. The first level of reform has to be at the grassroots level. This entails changing how anti-doping education is being imparted at the grassroots level. Further, the awareness level as to the rights of the athlete and the responsibility of the sports governing body has to be such that all stakeholders can make informed choices. Simplifying/ the language of the anti-doping programme and coordinating with the athletes' level of education is important. Using local language and dialect, in addition to the official language, is also important. This chapter will refer to other similar measures that need to be taken to protect the athletes from any systematic doping plan or inadvertent doping. At the second level, reform has to be vis-à-vis the International Federations and their role in implementing WADA. They have to collectively ensure that all of their officials and employees are effectively communicating with the athletes. Special focus has to be given to developing country athletes, ensuring better accessibility to both legal processes as well as forums for quick and just redressal of grievances. This chapter maps out the blueprint for doing the same. The third level has to be at the World Anti-Doping Agency and its Code. Functionally and structurally WADA has to have a more decentralized system, increasing accessibility for both athletes as well as officials of different countries. Increasing accountability and balancing it with the need to deter political pressure is the other challenge that needs to be addressed. Within the Code, substantial changes need to be made on issues of burden of proof, obtaining evidence and other methods for proving and sanctioning doping. On the whole, this chapter will propose a reform charter that urges a change in the present narrative.

Touching the ground – looking at the basics of anti-doping education

As the previous chapter showed, education on anti-doping issues needs to be emphasized. This is where the first structural reforms begin. The anti-doping awareness and education programme needs to be pushed up WADA's agenda as well as that of all the International Federations and the IOC. The content of the educational material should focus on the incentives of winning without doping. The focus needs to be shifted from the consequences of doping to the benefits of not doping. The target group of the anti-doping education and awareness programme will be varied, hence the focus and the content need to be customized. The current provision of anti-doping education and awareness in developing countries is not satisfactory. Countries like India continue to be bogged down with allegations of serious doping problems. The latest report published by WADA shows that India is amongst the top ten nations on the basis of doping violations. India holds the sixth position in terms of doping violations, which is an improvement. The last annual report published by WADA had placed India among the top three countries with the highest number of doping violations. NADA is happy with this improvement and takes the credit for an effective anti-doping awareness programme. Amongst the claims made by NADA was providing an e-learning facility.[1] However, a search on Google and repeated visits to NADA's website ended up being futile. No e-learning tab/portal was available on the NADA website. The anti-doping awareness programme should be less of a PR exercise and more of an effective anti-doping drive. The effectiveness can be increased only with an honest admission of the flaws.

A key feature of the anti-doping programme is that it has to be connected at the grassroots level. Hence, the materials that are distributed amongst the athletes need to be vetted. The more interesting the material, the more effective the message will be. The anti-doping education drive needs to cut down on the legal and scientific jargon that is in the Code. Any effective anti-doping programme has to speak the language of the target group. Stakeholders should put in an effort to simplify the terms and the concepts used in the anti-doping education drive. All the aspects of the current anti-doping programme, from sample collection, testing and result management to the finding of an ADRV should be explained in a language that is fathomable. In the developing country non-elite context, the language used has to reflect the emotions of the people being addressed. In the Indian context, for example, the rural and the urban divide has to be kept in mind. Similarly, the needs of junior- and school-level athletes differ from those of professional athletes. Hence, the anti-doping education and awareness programme cannot be the same for all. For a school-level athlete the programme

1 NADA, "WADA Report on Doping Violations: India Improves Its Global Anti-Doping Record" (2018) www.nadaindia.org/upload_file/document/1525277616.pdf (accessed 6 December 2018)

needs to focus more on the aspect of sport as a means to develop fitness, and the effect of drug abuse on the physiology. Similar to the good-touch, bad-touch lesson that children are taught in the context of child sexual abuse, a school-level athlete needs to be taught the good and the bad of anti-doping. Similarly, a junior-level athlete needs to be imparted with anti-doping education and awareness keeping in mind their concerns. Their needs will be more advanced than those of the school-level athletes.

When it comes to the non-elite professional athletes, who are the focus of this book, the approach has to be different. In the context of a developing country, the socio-cultural realities will have to be incorporated when designing the courses. The athletes' level of education also needs to be kept in mind. An illiterate non-elite professional athlete will be completely dependent on his or her coach for advice. Any effective anti-doping programme needs to first address this aspect of the coach–athlete relationship. The athlete needs to be assured of the checkpoints that are available in case the coach insists on consumption of food and nutritional supplements Or if the coach insists on designing their diet schedule and intake of medicines and so-called vitamin pills, the athlete should know where to cross check the coach's advice. The purpose is to ensure that the non-elite athlete feels empowered enough to make a decision independently. The anti-doping education and awareness programme needs to inform non-elite athletes of their rights. They should be informed that it has to be their choice to decide whether to ingest something or not. Athletes need to constantly question what things are being given to them as part of their training plan. Athletes need to be taught to respect but not to be subservient to their coach or any other official. The anti-doping programme in the context of developing countries needs to utilize the traditional means of mass entertainment to reach out to the athletes. For example, street plays, local theatre and folk songs could be used to make the non-elite athlete aware of the anti-doping programme.

Non-elite athletes need to be made computer- and tech-savvy. In the Indian context, for instance, NADA has not introduced any interactive videos through YouTube or other social media platforms. This is an important avenue which needs to be tapped into. Non-elite athletes could be reached through social network websites. Putting up videos and other interactive material would help keep the athletes informed. For example, each time a non-elite athlete logs into their social network account they would be able to access informational videos. For NADA, this would be a onetime investment with a repeat value. The anti-doping agencies of developing countries can overcome the constraints of budget allocation by using social media for educating their professional athletes. Seminars and workshops, unless they are interactive, become too academic and boring. These workshops should be designed to hold the non-elite athletes' attention. Apart from lawyers and scientists, such videos and workshops could feature sportspersons who are retired. These retired sportspersons could pass on their experiences of dealing with the system. For a non-elite athlete, the retired sportsperson acts as a role model. The non-elite athletes can learn a lot from the experiences of these role models. The effectiveness of these workshops and training programmes could be enhanced by conducting a mock trial with the help of the participants. The non-elite athletes can be made to retrace the steps that need to be taken to comply with the WADA system. The non-elite athletes also need to interact with coaches in an open forum so as to understand the nuances of a training programme that is in keeping with the requirements of the Code.

Coaches and the other support personnel should also be trained to design courses that keep in mind the socio-economic context. In the context of developing countries, coaches are often constrained because of the lack of resources. They need to be sensitized to the fact that shortcuts will not help them and resource constraints cannot be an excuse to use PEDs. The coaches need to be trained to be sensitive to the concerns of the athletes because the athletes come from a background where there is no exposure to anti-doping issues. The coaches need to understand that they are training professionals, and hence the transactions have to be above board. The training needs to be imparted to ensure that the coaches do not intimidate the non-elite athletes. The key to an effective awareness programme is transparency, trust and talk. Unless there is effective communication between the athlete and the coach, there will be no room for information sharing. The trust factor should not be treated as a means to override the opinion of the athlete. Coaches should be made to stay up-to-date with the developments taking place at the level of WADA. The coaches have to think not only in terms of winning but also in terms of compliance. Effort and energy need to be devoted to finding out alternative systems of training and diet plans sourced from local places. In the absence of world-class training facilities, coaches have to collectively put pressure on the government to invest in infrastructure development. Coaches have the vantage point to demand infrastructure improvements for they have the expertise. Using PEDs can thus not be treated as an alternative.

NADA also has the responsibility to make its booklet on WADA compliance more user-friendly. This is especially the case in the Indian context where the booklets currently available are mere pointers to the do's and don'ts. Detailed information based on the summary of the WADA anti-doping programme ought to be provided to the athletes. Further, NADA needs to promote transparency and awareness by designing different types of courses for different target groups. Considering the current standing of India amongst the most doped nations, steps urgently need to be taken. NADA needs to ensure transparency in result management and quick provision of hearings by the ADDP and the ADAP. The athletes need to be assured of a quick resolution of their disputes to instill certainty in the delivery of justice. Further, there needs to be constant communication between NADA and the National Federations in terms of effective awareness programmes and education. Any plan to effectively promote anti-doping awareness programmes needs to necessarily involve the athletes. For non-elite athletes there needs to be a feeling of participation in the anti-doping programme. Thus there needs to be a tripartite dialogue between NADA, the National Federation and the athlete. This dialogue also needs to include the athletes' support personnel.

Thus there needs to be an equal partnership between all the stakeholders viz. the athletes, the National Federations and NADA. Since the Indian government has a major role to play in the appointment of coaches, it needs to open avenues of interaction with the athletes on the problems they face. There has to be an athlete complaint redressal forum to enable the athletes to express their grievances. Finally, efforts need to be made in translating the complex WADA literature into as many local languages and dialects as possible. The wider and deeper the reach, the less chance of the non-elite being taken unaware. It will also empower the non-elite athlete to assess the dangers of consuming foods and other supplements. An effective anti-doping awareness programme at the grassroots level empowers the non-elite athlete to be an independent decision maker, and thus in a better position to negotiate the WADA mandate.

For NADA to do the above, governments will have to be proactive. NADA India for example is entirely government run. Hence, its effectiveness will be determined by the political will and commitment of the Indian government. As noted earlier, despite budget constraints, effective steps can be taken by doing the basics, such as the appointment of an independent person in charge of NADA and constituting an independent governing body. Governments should take a hands-off approach. The presence of government nominees and officials in the decision-making bodies of NADA creates a conflict of interest. The personal agenda of the government will come in direct conflict with the interest of the non-elite athlete. Considering that in India the government is also the job provider against the sports quota, there is a scenario of unequal bargaining power. Athletes cannot be expected to go against their employer, who is also in control of the anti-doping agency. Hence, structurally NADA India and similarly situated anti-doping agencies of developing countries ought to be outside the reach of government control. A model to emulate would be the Australian Sports Anti-Doping Agency (ASADA). Though financially and statutorily under the control of the Australian government, its organizational structure does not involve the interference of the government. Additionally, it has a dedicated department on legal and support services.[2] Considering the plight of the non-elite athlete from developing countries like India, providing legal support would go a long way in addressing their problems. The non-elite athletes of developing countries need to be elevated from the status of victims to that of policy influencers. And national governments do have an important role to play, for WADA can only issue guidelines at the international level. These guidelines have to be incorporated and implemented within the domestic legal framework by national governments. Logistical constraints notwithstanding, the basics of anti-doping framework viz. awareness and education need to be taken seriously.

2 Australian Sports Anti-Doping Agency, "Organisational Structure" www.asada.gov.au/sites/default/files/Org%20structure.pdf?v=1466401128 (accessed 5 December 2018)

The anti-doping programme and the International Federations – stop passing the buck!

On 2 July 2018, the Union Cycliste Internationale (UCI) issued a statement that "the anti-doping proceeding against Mr. Christopher Froome"[3] had been closed. Christopher Froome aka Chris Froome is a four-time Tour de France champion. He is one of the most recognized names amongst the current crop of pro cyclists. He is also the member of the wealthiest team in the professional cycling circuit.[4] This information is relevant in understanding the rationale behind the UCI's decision to drop anti-doping proceedings against its star cyclist. Froome was under doping suspicion since his sample tested for excess salbutamol. He was notified of the same during September 2017, after he won the Vuelta a España. It was during this competition that his sample was collected. The UCI took nine months to issue the above-quoted statement.[5] In the interim, the UCI initiated disciplinary proceedings, though no provisional suspension was imposed on Froome. His team supported him and did not ban him. Froome continued to win races during the nine months that the UCI was busy investigating him.[6] The use of salbutamol is permitted in a limited way viz. "Inhaled salbutamol: maximum 1600 micrograms over 24 hours in divided doses not to exceed 800 micrograms over 12 hours starting from any dose." Further, the WADA Prohibited List states that

> [t]he presence in urine of salbutamol in excess of 1000 ng/mL . . . is not consistent with therapeutic use of the substance and will be considered as an Adverse Analytical Finding (AAF) unless the Athlete proves, through a controlled pharmacokinetic study, that the abnormal result was the consequence of a therapeutic dose (by inhalation) up to the maximum dose indicated above.[7]

In Froome's case, the UCI struggled for nine months to arrive at a finding. The UCI accepted WADA's help to decipher the thousands of pages of documents that Froome and his team gave against the AAF argument. The UCI had both its and WADA's salbutamol experts to go through the evidence Froome produced.

3 Inside UCI, "UCI Statement on Anti-Doping Proceedings Involving Mr Christopher Froome" (2018) www.uci.org/inside-uci/press-releases/uci-statement-on-anti-doping-proceedings-involving-mr-christopher-froome (accessed 5 December 2018)

4 Joe Lindsey, "The Problem with Clearing Chris Froome the Uci's Decision Shows There Are Two Sets of Rules in Cycling: One for Rich Superstars, and One for Everyone Else" *Bicycling* (2018) www.bicycling.com/racing/a22038157/uci-chris-froome-doping/ (accessed 5 December 2018)

5 Inside UCI (n 3)

6 AFP/Bicycling.com, "Chris Froome Cleared in Doping Probe, Allowed to Race in Tour de France the Uci's Decision Clears Froome to Go for a Historic Fifth Tour Win" *Bicycling* (2018) www.bicycling.com/news/a22019610/chris-froome-cleared-doping/ (accessed 5 December 2018)

7 World Anti-Doping Code, "International Standard-Prohibited List" 1 January 2018 www.wada-ama.org/sites/default/files/prohibited_list_2018_en.pdf (accessed 6 December 2018)

The outcome of this review process showed that Froome had better research papers than WADA. On June 28 2018, WADA made the first move in this episode when it clarified to the UCI that "it would accept, based on the specific facts of the case, that Mr Froome's sample results do not constitute an AAF."[8] The UCI got the reprieve it was looking for to unburden itself and soon followed with the statement quoted at the beginning of this section. UCI justified the same saying that due to "WADA's unparalleled access to information and authorship of the salbutamol regime, the UCI has decided, based on WADA's position, to close the proceedings against Mr Froome."[9] The UCI sought to assure everyone that cycling was in good hands and that Froome had not been shown favouritism. The contradiction in this statement is revealed when on 6 July 2018 the UCI president went on record to state that "Froome had more financial support to find good experts to explain the situation."[10] This statement coming from the president of one of the leading International Sports Federations is telling. The UCI president also hinted at the possibility of riders placed similarly to Froome getting banned due to their inability to get the experts. The divide between elite and non-elite athletes, as argued in this book, once again was established. Indeed, there have been non-elite riders from developed countries who have been banned. Their salbutamol count was similar to that of Froome's. However, they had neither the star power nor the millions to challenge the UCI and WADA.[11]

This pro-elite approach was further evident when WADA, in defense of the Froome decision, justified the waiving of the controlled pharmacokinetic study. This study enables the athlete to re-enact the doses and the timings he used the salbutamol on the day of the test to rebut the charge of the AAF. If the sample used in the study returns the same result as on the day of the doping control, the athlete can successfully rebut the AAF.[12] This study is mandatory as per the 2018 WADA Prohibited List.[13] In Froome's case, WADA's statement in support of the waiver was

> It was accepted by the UCI, however, that in this case such a study would not have provided reliable evidence as it would be impossible to adequately recreate similar conditions to when Mr. Froome was subjected to the test, taking into account his physical condition, which included an illness, exacerbated asthmatic symptoms, dose escalation over a short period of time, dehydration and the fact that he was midway through a multi-day road cycling race.[14]

---

8 Inside UCI (n 3)

9 Ibid

10 Patrick Nathanson and Jack Skelton, "Chris Froome: UCI President Says Team Sky's Wealth Helped Them Fight Case in Way Other Teams Could Not" BBC *Sport* (London, 6 July 2018) www.bbc.com/sport/cycling/44739022 (accessed 5 December 2018)

11 Joe Lindsey (n 4)

12 Ibid

13 World Anti-Doping Code (n 7)

14 WADA, "WADA Clarifies Facts Regarding UCI Decision on Christopher Froome" (2018) www.wada-ama.org/en/media/news/2018-07/wada-clarifies-facts-regarding-uci-decision-on-christopher-froome (accessed 5 December 2018)

One would assume that such exemptions have been granted to all who were similarly exhausted due to a tough road cycling race. The facts though reveal a different picture. Froome is the lucky one to have been bestowed with such a privilege.[15] The UCI denies any such favouritism and wants people to forget the past and look to the future. The future however does not appear to be bright. The conduct of the UCI may not be indicative of the fact that all the International Federations are pro-elite; however, there is hardly any evidence to the contrary where stars are hauled up without being egged on by the public opinion. As was seen in the case of the Russian scandal, the IAAF's former president Lamine Diack was involved in the cover-up in lieu of money.[16] Thus, the International Federations have been instrumental in skewing the anti-doping enforcement against the non-elites.

As the Froome case reveals, if the non-elite of the First World can feel left out and discriminated against, the plight of the non-elite of the developing world is even worse. The power of money appears to rule the roost, and the UCI's past proves the statement true. The Lance Armstrong case is a classic example of how the elite stars of the sports world can con the anti-doping system. Lance Armstrong was a seven-time Tour de France champion from 1999 to 2005. He continues to hold the record for the most wins by any cyclist in the history of the championship.[17] One cannot get more elite than that. An Armstrong doping win, when discovered, was regarded as "more extensive than any previously revealed in professional sports history."[18] He won all seven titles with the help of PEDs and was a supplier of the same to his teammates. He ensured, because of his dominance within the team, that everyone else used PEDs as well. Like his sporting career, in terms of doping violations, too, he can be regarded as one of the most decorated. Armstrong was sanctioned for

(1) Use and/or attempted use of prohibited substances and/or methods including EPO, blood transfusions, testosterone, corticosteroids and/or masking agents.

(2) Possession of prohibited substances and/or methods including EPO, blood transfusions and related equipment (such as needles, blood bags, storage containers and other transfusion equipment and blood parameters measuring devices), testosterone, corticosteroids and/or masking agents

15 Joe Lindsey (n 4)
16 SI Wire, "Ex-IAAF President Lamine Diack Confesses to Asking Russia for Money" *Sports Illustrated* (2015) www.si.com/more-sports/2015/12/18/iaaf-corruption-lamine-diack-confession-russian-doping-scandal-bribe (accessed 5 December 2018)
17 "Lance Armstrong Stripped of All Seven Tour de France Wins by UCI" BBC (London, 22 October 2012) www.bbc.com/sport/cycling/20008520 (accessed 5 December 2018)
18 United States Anti-Doping Agency, "United States Anti-Doping Agency, Claimant, v. Lance Armstrong, Respondent-reasoned Decision of the United States Anti-Doping Agency on Disqualification and Ineligibility" (2012) Report on Proceedings Under the World Anti-Doping Code and the Usada Protocol

(3) Trafficking of EPO, testosterone, and/or corticosteroids

(4) Administration and/or attempted administration to others of EPO, testosterone, and/or cortisone

(5) Assisting, encouraging, aiding, abetting, covering up and other complicity involving one or more anti-doping rule violations and/or attempted anti-doping rule violations

(6) Aggravating circumstances (including multiple rule violations and participated in a sophisticated scheme and conspiracy to dope, encourage and assist others to dope and cover up rule violations) justifying a period of ineligibility greater than the standard sanction.[19]

The USADA was able to detect Armstrong's doping programme through the whistle-blowing and assistance provided by his former teammates.[20] Armstrong initially denied the charges of doping and tried to get a stay against the USADA sanctions by filing a lawsuit in the US District Court of Texas. However, the District Court refused to intervene. Hence, Armstrong was left with no choice but to challenge the finding of the USADA before neutral arbitrators or face sanctions for doping. Armstrong decided not to challenge the sanctions before neutral arbitrators.[21] Accordingly, the USADA proceeded to give its reasoned decision supporting sanctioning against Armstrong. The USADA found that

1   Armstrong used PED EPO.

2   He used testosterone.

3   He supplied PEDs to his teammates.

4   He personally administered PEDs to his teammates.

5   He coerced his teammates to take PEDs with the threat of termination from the team.

6   Dr Michele Ferrari was the author of the systematic doping program.

7   Armstrong used the services of Dr Ferrari for implementing the doping program.

8   Armstrong forced his teammates to use the services of Dr Ferrari.[22]

The USADA reasoned that the evidence against Armstrong was strong enough to prove his doping beyond a reasonable doubt. Armstrong's ADRV was proven through non-analytical evidence based on witness statements. The USADA therefore reasoned that Armstrong's ADRV stood proven.[23] As per the witness account, Armstrong had been using EPO since 1998, while making his mark on the tour circuit. Armstrong also ensured that his teammates used EPO. It was

19 Ibid 8–9
20 Ibid 10
21 Ibid 12–13
22 Ibid
23 Ibid 15–16

also during the same time that Armstrong was using cortisone.[24] This is ironic because 1998 was also the year the Festina scandal took place. This is a good example of the failure of the International Federations to take any effective steps even after a series of scandals hit the sport. The Armstrong case also revealed that Armstrong and his support staff manipulated the UCI system, smuggling PEDs in right under their noses.[25] Armstrong drew up a detailed plan to win the Tour de France and avoid getting detected. As the USADA report notes, "First, the UCI had no organized out of competition testing program," hence Armstrong could not be caught in the run up to the Tour. "Second . . . as there existed no whereabouts program that required riders to provide their training location for testing . . . the prospect of unannounced testing was even more remote," since Armstrong used to train in remote locations. "Third, the sheer length and severity of the Tour de France greatly increases the pay off of doping. A rider doping in the Tour has an even greater advantage over non-doping competitors than in a shorter competition."[26]

WADA was non-existent when Armstrong devised his plan to con the system. Interestingly, however, Armstrong's doping practices were detected only in 2012 through non-analytical evidence. Further, WADA came into existence in the year 1999 and the WADA Code came into force in 2004. Additionally, the Code underwent revisions and the revised version came into force in 2009. In between all these measures Armstrong continued to dope and win. He was able to not only exploit the naïve WADA-run system of 2004 but also the experienced anti-doping system of 2009.

The revisions were made to make the system more stringent, compliances more onerous and life more difficult for the non-elite developing country athletes. Armstrong, on the other hand, used the advantages of his elite, powerful status to customize the outcomes of the anti-doping programme. Hence the legitimacy of the system and the willpower of the International Federations is debatable. In the sports hierarchy, the International Federations have the most important role to play because they dictate the rules and regulations to the National Federations. Hence it is important that they scrutinize their National Federations and ensure accountability. Hence, the laxity and faults within the UCI system that Armstrong used to his advantages put strain on any scope of accountability amongst the sports authorities. Armstrong's US Postal Service team facilitated his mission to win a record number of Tour de France titles.[27] The amazing bit was that Armstrong was able to hoodwink the tight security put into place during the Tour de France to ensure uninterrupted supplies of the PEDs.[28] Armstrong's performance created quite a surprise when he won the Tour in such a dominating

24 Ibid 18–19
25 Ibid 20
26 Ibid 21–22
27 Ibid 28
28 Ibid 30

manner. The effect of his successful PEDs programme was on display. However, there was no one who could devise a way of catching him off-guard.[29] Armstrong further manipulated the system by adding blood doping to his menu. The USADA report states:

> The reinfused blood would boost the oxygen carrying capacity of Armstrong's blood and that of his lieutenants and help their stamina and ability to recover. . . . There was no test for blood transfusions, so this method of cheating would be undetectable. . . . The whole process took about an hour and then it was time for Armstrong and his teammates to do a training ride down the coast. . . . After having lost a bag of blood Armstrong, Hamilton and Livingston were all "quickly fatigued." Three elite-level athletes who were regarded as among the best cyclists in the world "could barely make it up small hills." Once the blood was re-infused, however, the cyclists' climbing power would be greatly enhanced.[30]

The French investigators were suspicious and initiated a doping investigation against Armstrong and his team. As expected, there were denials, and there was no proof that could lead to any findings of doping. This was the case with every suspicion and every accusation made against Armstrong each time he won the Tour.[31] As the USADA documents, Armstrong confidently told lies about never doping. The USADA portrays Armstrong's conduct not as that of a sportsperson, but as that of a calm and cool criminal having no qualms about doing anything in order to win.[32] The USADA documents the fact that despite Dr Michele Ferrari being under investigation for doping Armstrong continued his association.[33] Later when Dr Ferrari was convicted for sporting fraud and distribution of doping products and devising doping plans for athletes, Armstrong went into PR overdrive.[34] Armstrong issued a public statement disassociating himself from Dr Ferrari. However when it came to winning his seventh Tour title, he, as per the USADA, resumed his partnership with Ferrari.[35] The USADA thus documented the series of events and circumstantial evidence needed to establish Armstrong's ADRV. In addition, Armstrong's refusal to testify before the USADA was also regarded as an ADRV,[36] as per Article 3.2.4 of the 2009 WADA Code.[37] There

29 Ibid 34–35
30 Ibid 39
31 Ibid 42–43
32 Ibid 45
33 Ibid 68
34 Ibid 73–74
35 Ibid 77
36 Ibid 87–88
37 WADA 2009, Article 3.2.4 [The hearing panel in a hearing on an anti-doping rule violation may draw an inference adverse to the Athlete or other Person who is asserted to have committed an anti-doping rule violation based on the Athlete's or other Person's refusal, after a request made

was evidence, as per the USADA, to implicate Armstrong's support staff for doping.[38] Armstrong and his team were found by the USADA to have successfully avoided testing positive. That, too, was part of the sophisticated plan developed over the years.[39] Finally, the USADA had the blood samples collected from Armstrong re-analysed. Using better testing methods, the results of re-analyses provided evidence of blood doping.[40]

In this case the USADA sought and was successful in getting all of Armstrong's competitive results annulled from 1998 on.[41] For the same, the USADA determined that the eight-year limitation period as given in the 2009 WADA Code stood suspended.[42] As per the USADA:

> The eight-year statute of limitation found in Article 17 of the Code was suspended by Mr. Armstrong's fraudulent concealment of his doping. In asserting anti-doping rule violations and disqualifying results older than the eight year limitation period found in Article 17 of the Code, USADA is relying on the well-established principle that the running of a statute of limitation is suspended when the person seeking to assert the statute of limitation defense has subverted the judicial process, such as by fraudulently concealing his wrongful conduct.[43]

The USADA concluded its investigation and report with a clear finding of ADRVs and statement on imposition of sanction. As per the USADA, the sanction would be disqualification of results and imposition of ineligibility for life. The Armstrong saga was thus brought to an end by the USADA. What is missing from the above narrative is the UCI. The USADA documented the ineptness of the UCI as a story of denial of the existence of doping. Armstrong was the UCI's star and crowd puller. The UCI refused to believe that Armstrong had used PEDs. The USADA documents that

> UCI has never claimed it discovered any violation based on the Landis email, but instead has always contended the email was not evidence of anything and sued Landis for defamation based on its content. Not surprisingly, then,

---

in a reasonable time in advance of the hearing, to appear at the hearing (either in person or telephonically as directed by the hearing panel) and to answer questions from the hearing panel or the Anti-Doping Organization asserting the anti-doping rule violation.]
38 United States Anti-Doping Agency (n 18) 90
39 Ibid 134–135
40 Ibid 141
41 Ibid 154
42 WADA 2009, Article 17 [Article 17: Statute of Limitations-No action may be commenced against an Athlete or other Person for an anti-doping rule violation contained in the Code unless such action is commenced within eight (8) years from the date the violation is asserted to have occurred.]
43 United States Anti-Doping Agency (n 18) 154

UCI did not initiate any investigation based on the Landis email. Indeed, UCI has consistently stated (as recently as July 2012) that it is unable to determine whether or not an antidoping violation has occurred. 833 UCI cannot claim, on the one hand, that it discovered the violations, while on the other hand taking the position it still does not know whether any violation occurred. Finally, during a videotaped interview conducted on July 11, 2012, UCI's President, Pat McQuaid, stated that UCI is "not involved in this, it's a USADA investigation," and that "it's nothing to do with UCI, and [UCI] will wait and see what the eventual outcome is."[44]

Continuing further with the story of the inaction of UCI, the USADA stated that

> In 2010 when Mr. Landis publicly raised his allegations of Mr. Armstrong's doping, in an Associated Press article UCI President McQuaid responded before undertaking any investigation whatsoever, contending that Mr. Landis' allegations in his April 30, 2010 email were "nothing new" and that, "he already made those accusations in the past." Rather than investigate the allegations, instead the UCI sued Mr. Landis. Similarly, when Tyler Hamilton publicly explained his knowledge of Mr. Armstrong's doping in a 60 Minutes interview nationally telecast in the United States and reported around the world in May, 2011, the UCI's Honorary President and current UCI Management Committee Member, Hein Verbruggen, stated: That's impossible, because there is nothing. I repeat again: Lance Armstrong has never used doping. Never, never, never. And I say this not because I am a friend of his, because that is not true. I say it because I'm sure.[45]

Need one say more about how the International Federation reacted and played out its responsibility to be vigilant? Armstrong implicitly was allowed free run because the UCI chose to look the other way while doping was going on. The statements issued by the UCI during the Armstrong investigation have an uncanny similarity to the statements issued by the UCI during the Froome investigation. It means that any structural reforms urging the International Federations to get their house in order and pull up their socks are bound to fall flat. The measures of taking timely action, of initiating fair and transparent investigations of applying rules transparently to everyone are things that do not take much effort. There needs to be the will to look at sports as an activity involving the livelihood of all viz. the elite as well as the non-elite. If there is going to be favouritism towards the elite and persecution of the non-elite, the developing countries' non-elite will be done for good. They have to give up hope of being treated fairly under the

44 Ibid 159
45 Ibid 160

stringent anti-doping regime. As mentioned earlier, the more onerous 2009 Code did not ruffle Armstrong's feathers but has definitely affected the non-elite developing countries athletes. It has made their lives more difficult and their chance of practicing and competing in sports without fear more remote.

Ashamed at the occurrence of the Armstrong doping scandal, which matched the Festina scandal in terms of shock value, the UCI constituted the Cycling Independent Reform Commission (CIRC). It submitted its report on February 2015. The CIRC was constituted to

> conduct a wide-ranging independent investigation to establish the roots, historical reasons, causes, mechanisms, processes, procedures, practices, patterns, networks, providers, instigators and facilitators that enabled the endemic problem of doping in cycling.
>
> To investigate whether UCI officials directly contributed to the development of a culture of doping in cycling, in particular by mismanaging the testing and/or by covering up positive tests, and whether the UCI and other governing bodies and officials were implicated in ineffective investigation of doping practices.
>
> To produce a report at the end of the CIRC mandate for the President of the UCI, that provides knowledge and understanding of the past endemic culture of doping in cycling, and provides targeted recommendations to the whole cycling community for the future.[46]

The findings of the report affirmed the statement of the USADA as quoted above. The CIRC report confirmed that Lance Armstrong was given preferential treatment. There was a waiver of the mandatory rules in Armstrong's case. Anti-doping compliances were thus relaxed for Armstrong. The justification for the same is Armstrong's status as the star cyclist. The CIRC noted that

> UCI saw Lance Armstrong as the perfect choice to lead the sport's renaissance after the Festina scandal: the fact that he was American opened up a new continent for the sport, he had beaten cancer and the media quickly made him a global star.[47]

The UCI had a crisis in its internal governance, with the president having immense power. The system also lacked effective checks and balances. Consequently, there were issues of governance and a lack of transparency. Doping in cycling therefore was seen by the UCI as an irritant which was contained to harp on the image of a clean sport. As in the Armstrong case, rules were not strictly imposed and issues

---

46 Cycling Independent Reform Commission, *Report to the President of the Union Cycliste Internationale* (2015) *Lausanne* 16 https://s27394.pcdn.co/wp-content/uploads/2015/03/CIRC-Report-2015.pdf (accessed 3 December 2018)

47 Ibid 7

were pushed under the carpet. However, as pointed out, the UCI tweaked the rules only to promote the interests of its elite athletes. Protecting the interests of the elites meant protecting the commercial interest of the sport. Thus, there were no strong anti-doping measures.[48] Things changed with the growing clamour for action. Sponsors and broadcasters mounted pressure to clean up the system. The UCI devised more effective anti-doping enforcement policies post 2006/2007.[49] The CIRC noted that UCI had created an independent Cycling Anti-Doping Foundation (CADF).[50] However, the leadership continued to interfere with anti-doping enforcement. Hence, the changes notwithstanding, poor governance meant that elites continued to get away with manipulating the system. As per the CIRC:

> The general view is that at the elite level the situation has improved, but that doping is still taking place. . . . In contrast to the findings in previous investigations, which identified systematic doping organised by teams, at the elite level riders who dope now organise their own doping programmes with the help of third parties who are primarily outside the cycling team. At the elite level, doping programmes are generally sophisticated and therefore doctors play a key role in devising programmes that provide performance enhancement whilst minimising the risk of getting caught. . . . Factors still exist that could be seen to encourage or facilitate doping. For example: there is financial instability throughout the sport (teams often depend entirely on one sponsor, and teams, and therefore riders, can be under huge pressure to obtain good results to keep sponsors or get an extension of their short-term contract).[51]

As could be seen in Froome's case, the elite will continue to exploit the system. The CIRC acknowledged the advantages that elites and rich cyclists have over the non-elite teams and athletes. Accordingly, its recommendations largely centred around the issues of a fair and transparent system of governance being in place. The CIRC recommended that

1   The sports governing bodies are to be responsible for carrying out anti-doping measures. However, they are to work closely with governments to deal with law-and-order issues, including criminal investigations.
2   The doctors found to have been involved in doping infractions should also be reported to their regulatory bodies in order to be barred from general medical practice.
3   The sports governing bodies should be bound by confidentiality clauses. Accordingly, the culture of naming and shaming with respect to doping allegations should be avoided until the investigations are completed.

---

48 Ibid 9
49 Ibid 52
50 Ibid 11
51 Ibid 12

4   The UCI and its anti-doping agency should conduct wide-ranging studies
     to find out the extent of doping. The investigations ought to be carried out
     across different countries and groups viz. amateur and professional. Such a
     study, as per the CIRC, would enable the UCI to utilize its resources in an
     efficient way and avoid waste of effort.
5   The UCI/CADF should conduct qualitative instead of quantitative analy-
     ses. Further testing should be conducted based on the information received.
     The UCI ought to rely on non-analytical evidence to target individual
     riders and support staff. The tests are to be both in- and out-of-competition
     tests.
6   A well-developed system to re-test and re-analyse samples would be an effec-
     tive measure against doping. A sample, once given, should be able to be re-
     tested based on the availability of better scientific tools. Thus, retrospective
     testing is recommended as integral part of doping control.
7   An effective whistle-blowing scheme should be put in place. The whistle-
     blower desk has to be independent so as to instill confidence and inspire
     whistle-blowers to come forward with information. In addition, the UCI is
     advised to make full use of the substantial assistance scheme. Consequently,
     all International Federations have the liberty to re-analyse the samples to
     find out about past infractions.

The CIRC's recommendation also dealt with governance and education issues.
CIRC thus recommended that

> UCI carry out a study on the election process to make it more transpar-
> ent, democratic, representative and straightforward, perhaps to include
> voting rights for representatives of professional licence holders. CIRC
> considers that past elections for president were seriously flawed and
> lessons should be learned from those past mistakes.
> Checks and balances
> The Commission considers that there should be better control and
> accountability for UCI in the form of its overarching management
> body, which has effective financial control over all actions, commis-
> sions and bodies of UCI.
> CIRC recommends that the Ethics Commission should be revamped to
> ensure it is independently appointed and that people who are cited
> are obliged to cooperate. The Ethics Commission should be proactive
> rather than reactive. Furthermore, the Ethics Commission's mandate
> should not be linked to the president's term in office, so that it cannot
> be dissolved immediately after an election.
> CIRC recommends that Management Committee members should take
> a more active role and be accountable. CIRC also recommends that,
> unlike in the past, everything that occurs during committee meetings
> should be recorded in the minutes . . .

> The CIRC recommends using sanctioned riders as an educational tool. This should include interviews with the rider, appearances, lectures and recorded messages pointing out the impact of doping on their lives. The information should detail the social stigma, financial impact, health effects and self-esteem issues. UCI should be creative and make the education programme relevant to young athletes through the use of social media . . .
>
> CIRC recommends that if competitions are devised in which teams of different tour levels are competing, that all teams are subject to the same level of testing, and always to the higher standard.
>
> CIRC recommends that UCI take steps to address the lack of financial stability for teams and riders, which currently fosters an environment that pushes teams and riders to do all they can to achieve results.[52]

The CIRC report thus does not provide any innovative or out-of-the-box ideas to reform the UCI. However, it does recommend the basics that are expected of any International Federation. One such requirement is to apply all the rules equally to all athletes. Practically, if that is not done, then there is no scope of reform. Access to resources like better awareness programmes is on the usual lines. The UCI has since then not had any major scandals to deal with, though suspicion continues to linger as to the current state of affairs. The UCI is trying to stringently coordinate with WADA on anti-doping enforcement. The example of the UCI is nonetheless revealing of the prevailing attitude of the leading International Federation of the sport. And with corruption running through the highest level of governance and management, the scope of implementing genuine and far-reaching reforms is not easy to come by.

The IAAF's role in the Russian doping scandal is a good example of how the International Federations have the ability to pick and choose the method of anti-doping enforcement. If the target group is potentially rich and influential, norms will be scuttled. And it is not just the UCI and IAAF that have promoted the elite agenda. The other sports giant, FIFA, has also been found wanting when it comes to applying rules properly and stringently.

A report published in Spiegel Online alleges that Sergio Ramos, captain of both Real Madrid and the Spanish National Team, tested positive for the use of PED. However, this was never reported and acted upon. No investigation has been initiated nor have any of the mandated steps under WADA, post positive test, been taken. The report implicates the Union of European Football Associations (UEFA) for complicity and cover up. Ramos is regarded as one of the best football players in the world, having won the World Cup once, the European championship twice and a three-time Champions League winner.[53] Ramos

52 Ibid 220–223
53 Der Spiegel Staff, "Doping Irregularities Ramos, Ronaldo and the Controllers" *Spiegel Online* (Berlin, 23 November 2018) www.spiegel.de/international/world/football-leaks-doping-tests-and-real-madrid-a-1240035.html (accessed 4 December 2018)

belongs to the elite of football players, and hence the allegations are another example of a pro-elite stand.

To buttress its argument of discrimination in favour of the elite of football, the report cites another incident involving Cristiano Ronaldo. The report alleges that during an unannounced doping control, Ronaldo objected to the doping control officer taking his sample. Further, Real Madrid, the team to which Ronaldo belongs, sent its own medical personnel to complete the collection of the sample.[54] Such interventions are fundamentally against the idea of free and fair anti-doping measures. The report once again points to the complicity of the UEFA, given that it went along with the interference of Real Madrid in the sample collection and doping control process. Considering, that the UEFA is in charge of result management in connection with the UEFA Champions League, this is a serious allegation and proves lack of independence.

Another instance cited in the report points out that Ramos refused to cooperate with the Spanish Anti-Doping Agency during the doping control. However, no action has been initiated, and the matter is closed.[55]

The truth of the matter is that unless the International Federations are pro-active the elites will get away with anti-doping violations. This is because the current structures within international sports are modelled on the principle of conflict of interest. There cannot be any possible independent entity, without an agenda, sincerely implementing the rules. Again, India can be cited as a case in point. In India, although all sportspersons are amenable to the jurisdiction of the NADA, the cricketers are outside its ambit. Accordingly, all sportspersons except cricketers are required to stringently comply with the WADA Code. The Board of Control for Cricket in India (BCCI) has vehemently rejected all efforts to bring it under the aegis of the NADA, being a national sports governing body, but to date all such efforts have been futile.[56] The point being made is that in the world of sport there are two systems: one for the elite and the other for the non-elite. BCCI is the most powerful sports governing body in India. Accordingly, it does not depend on the state to fund its activities. Therefore, it continues to defy the dictate of the state and WADA. Further, cricket is not an Olympic sport, and hence the BCCI need not bother with complying with the WADA Code as a pre-condition to participating in the Olympics. The cricketers are thus grouped into the class of elite sportspersons, though they belong to a developing country. The plight of the non-elite athlete continues unabated and they are required to stringently comply with the WADA Code. This discussion thus underlines the fact that in some instances the national governing body is so powerful that the International Federation has to bow to its demands. In the context of the BCCI,

54 Ibid
55 Ibid
56 TNN, "BCCI Turns Down Wada's Demand to Test Cricketers" *The Times of India Sports* (New Delhi, 11 November 2017) https://timesofindia.indiatimes.com/sports/cricket/news/bcci-turns-down-wadas-demand-to-test-cricketers/articleshow/61601043.cms (accessed 4 December 2018)

the International Cricket Council (ICC) is subservient to the BCCI. The ICC has been a WADA signatory since 2006, however it neither has the willpower nor the bargaining power to deal with the BCCI.

As a cricketing powerhouse the BCCI provides the lifeblood of international cricket viz. money and spectators. The BCCI provides the largest share of fans and the biggest chunk of revenue to the ICC.[57] In the absence of the BCCI, the ICC's survival would be at stake. This is probably a rare case of an International Federation being weaker than the National Federation. Broadcasters look to the BCCI to generate television and other broadcasting revenue. In such a scenario, the ICC will never force the BCCI to be Code compliant. Hence, in all BCCI-organized matches, national or international, WADA will have no applicability. This is the reality of sports. Transparency, accountability and equality are all words and mere words in the field of sports. The non-elites of developing countries will continue to suffer unless the will to take on the might of financial behemoths is there amongst all. Considering that there are other members in the ICC like Australia, South Africa, England and so on, their silence in obliging to the BCCI is surprising. If they had the political will they would have collectively acted against the BCCI and would have forced the BCCI to implement the WADA Code and impose the same on its cricketers. It appears though that no one is willing to upset the apple cart. Since revenue generation appears to be the most important agenda of all the International Federations, no one is interested in ensuring implementation of the anti-doping norms.

Hence, the blueprint for addressing the developing countries' concerns lies in changing the attitudes of the International Federations. The preference of commercial over other interests is the biggest hindrance for any positive change. As the CIRC report notes, the International Federations are to ensure that the rules are applied to all. There should not be any waiver or relaxation in compliance procedure in favour of any specific athlete. The non-elite athlete's concerns should be addressed by ensuring that the National Federations in the developing country develop sensitization programmes on anti-doping issues. The International Federations should constantly monitor that the National Federations are complying with their mandate and discharging their responsibilities. The International Federations should insist that National Federations have a legal advisory office to deal with the legal issues that are associated with anti-doping enforcement. The International Federations need to provide a forum for interactions between different stakeholders about the difficulties they are facing. Hence, the IFs should require the National Federations to develop outreach programmes for their athletes designed to make them understand the anti-doping regime. Athletes should have ease of access to the officeholders and the decision makers

---

57 A L I Chougule, "BCCI Must Go Easy on Muscle-flexing" *The Free Press Journal* (New Delhi, 12 May 2017) www.freepressjournal.in/editorspick/ali-chougule-bcci-must-go-easy-on-muscle-flexing/1066668 (accessed 6 December 2018)

within the National Federations. The International Federations have the power to de-recognize the National Federations. Hence, complying with anti-doping education and awareness programmes should be criteria for recognizing or de-recognizing a National Federation. International Federations can also consult with the national governments of developing countries to develop effective programmes to ensure that they are able to deal with the WADA-run anti-doping programme. Partnering with both National Federations and national governments can also help in dealing with legal issues such as drug trafficking. Further, the International Federations should provide the National Federations of developing countries with funds to be used for the enhancement of athlete welfare. The International Federations should also work towards technology transfer in terms of advanced training facilities to empower the developing country non-elite athlete. On the whole, engaging with the National Federation and the non-elite developing country athlete is key to an inclusive approach. It will ensure that the athletes do not feel discriminated against compared to the rich and powerful. It will also ensure that the non-elite athlete is better equipped to handle any legal challenge. Further, doping-related disputes need to be quickly handled by the National Federations. Accordingly, the National Federations should work with NADA to bring about quick redressal.

Structural reforms within WADA? A distant dream

Within WADA there are several key areas on which one can argue for reforms. Substantively there are areas which need to be revisited. The WADA 2021 Code revision process has been initiated and remains ongoing. It is an apt moment to reflect upon the possible revisions to the 2015 Code that should be incorporated and put into effect. Accordingly, WADA has initiated discussion on a set of questions without touching upon the basic philosophical aspects of WADA. Thus issues like strict liability, burden of proof and proof of ADRVs through non-analytical methods are all outside the scope of review. The following issues have been opened for review:

1 Expansion of the categories of doping as given under Article 2.
2 Presumption of the validity of WADA Decision Limit in the same way as WADA's Prohibited List.
3 Expanding the base of athletes who need to submit to whereabouts requirements.
4 Re-analyses of samples and resolving the question of ownership of samples.
5 Resolving the issue of overlapping authority in result management.
6 Issues pertaining to the reduction/elimination of sanctions due to consumption of contaminated food supplements, especially through meat consumption.
7 Debate on the desirable standard that needs to be followed when proving the source of a prohibited substance.

8   Clarifying the standards that need to be looked into to prove No-Significant Fault/Negligence.
9   Issue of burden of proof in the case of a minor.
10   Changing the scope of multiple violations and what should be regarded as such.
11   In case of delays in investigation and disposal of appeals, who should bear the burden.
12   Further strengthening the notification process and appeal process.
13   Addressing privacy and data protection issues.
14   Automatic recognition of sanctions by all signatories.
15   Developing international standards pertaining to education and awareness of the anti-doping programme.
16   Accountability of all the officials involved in anti-doping enforcement.
17   Obligation on the national anti-doping agency to investigate at the direction of WADA.
18   Enhancing capabilities to effectively track athlete support personnel.
19   Revising laboratory accreditation standards.
20   Compliance issues of the signatories including the roles and responsibilities of WADA need to be debated.
21   Developing stringent rules to ensure Code compliance and incorporate clearly defined consequences for non-compliance.
22   Relooking at the issue of governance within WADA.
23   Debating the outsourcing of work to third-party anti-doping service providers.
24   Recognition and protection of whistle-blowers.[58]

These points aside, WADA needs to include the abuse of technology to enhance performance. The use of a light weight bat or cycle or advanced shoes are some of the examples of how technology can be abused. Though equipment specifications are laid down by the International Federations, elite athletes have access to advanced scientific research and the opportunity to manipulate the same.[59] The CIRC report did refer to such infractions.[60] The incorporation of such a provision will go a long way in addressing one concern of the non-elite athlete from a developing country, which is lack of access to advanced technology. Further WADA should, as part of its standard of education and awareness, insist on the sharing

58 WADA, "2021 World Anti-Doping Code Review: Questions to Discuss and Consider" As Per the Decision Taken by the WADA Foundation Board on 16 November 2017 in Seoul, Korea www.wada-ama.org/sites/default/files/2021codereview_questions.pdf (accessed 5 December 2018)
59 Bryce Dyer, "The Controversy of Sports Technology: A Systematic Review" SpringerPlus (2015) www.ncbi.nlm.nih.gov/pmc/articles/PMC4575312/ (accessed 4 December 2018)
60 Xataka, "Everything About Technological Doping in Cycling" Medium (2015) https://medium.com/@Xataka/everything-about-technological-doping-in-cycling-78c7fd1fe3f   (accessed   5   December 2018)

of research output on training modules. There should be a specific provision, as part of its role and responsibility, that WADA should monitor effective technology transfer from the developed to the developing countries. Lack of adequate training facilities has hampered the careers of thousands of non-elite developing country athletes. Their capabilities have not been enhanced due to the dearth of resources. Hence when it comes to ensuring fairness in sport, training equipment and access to technology needs to form part of the discourse. WADA being the one dealing with compliances of anti-doping measures should ensure that no one gains any advantage in any artificial way whatsoever. WADA is expanding its Prohibited List and adding newer substances and methods. Technology doping and non-transfer of advanced technology to non-elite developing country athletes should be regarded as an ADRV.

That WADA is dictated by the sentiments of the international community is evident from its reaction to the recent decision of the European Court of Human Rights (ECHR). On 18 January 2018, the ECHR gave its ruling on a number of applications that challenged the validity of whereabouts requirements.[61] The challenges arose from the act of the French government amending its Sports Code to make it WADA compliant. Consequently, the amendment incorporated the whereabouts compliance requirement in tune with the WADA Code and International Standards. The applicants, who all were athletes belonging to different sports organizations, arg Though the committee did not address the issue, lack of trained support personnel and anti-doping education means that athletes in India also do not have access to adequate legal advice. ued that the whereabouts requirement within the French Sports Code violated their rights as protected under Article 8 of the European Convention on Human Rights.[62] They argued that

> With regard to the whereabouts requirement provided for in those Articles, they complained of a "particularly intrusive" testing system which compelled athletes in the testing pool to provide the AFLD with information concerning their places of residence, training and competition so that they could be located at any time, and to undergo immediate tests ordered on a discretionary basis and without advance notice. They complained in particular of the fact that the tests could be carried out independently of sporting events and

61 National Federation of Sportspersons' Associations and Unions (FNASS) and Others V. France ECHR (Fifth Section) 2018 https://hudoc.echr.coe.int/eng#{%22itemid%22:[%22001-180442%22]} (accessed 6 December 2018)

62 European Convention on Human Rights, Article 8 [Right to respect for private and family life 1. Everyone has the right to respect for his private and family life, his home and his correspondence. 2. There shall be no interference by a public authority with the exercise of this right except such as is in accordance with the law and is necessary in a democratic society in the interests of national security, public safety or the economic well-being of the country, for the prevention of disorder or crime, for the protection of health or morals, or for the protection of the rights and freedoms of others] www.echr.coe.int/Documents/Convention_ENG.pdf (accessed 7 December 2018)

outside training periods, that is . . . [they] were on holiday, resting or on sick leave or leave following an occupational injury. They argued that Article 3 infringed their freedom of movement by requiring them to give notice of their whereabouts on an ongoing basis, including during non-professional activities, and also infringed their right to a normal family life and their individual freedom as athletes.[63]

In their view, the unconditional implementation of Article 3(I)(3)(d) of the Order, allowing tests to be carried out independently of sporting events and outside training periods, meant that between 6 a.m. and 9 p.m. (the testing period laid down by Article L. 232–14 of the Sports Code, see paragraph 64 below) the athletes in the testing pool faced the permanent prospect of physically intrusive tests. This entailed systematically giving advance notice of their schedule, in breach of the right to establish relationships with their peers and the right to the peaceful enjoyment of their private lives. Lastly, the applicants complained of a breach of the principle of equality, as the whereabouts requirement for the purposes of anti-doping tests was confined to athletes included in the testing pool.[64]

The French Supreme Court Conseil d'Éta rejected these arguments and upheld the validity of whereabouts on the basis that

These provisions provide a strict framework . . . They require the athletes in question, in view of the demands of efforts to combat doping, to provide accurate and up-to-date information on their whereabouts for the purposes of organising tests, including unannounced tests, with a view to the effective detection of the use of doping substances. . . . Hence, Articles 3 and 7 of the impugned order, which do not hamper athletes' freedom of movement, interfere with their right to respect for their private and family life as guaranteed by Article 8, and with individual freedoms, only to the extent that is necessary and proportionate to the general-interest aims pursued by efforts to combat doping, namely to protect athletes' health and to ensure fair and ethical sporting competitions.

The principle of equality does not prevent the regulatory authority from laying down different rules for different situations or from derogating from equality on general interest grounds, provided that, in both cases, the resulting difference in treatment is proportionate to the purpose of the rule establishing it.[65]

These provisions provide a strict framework governing the locations where AFLD testing of athletes in the "testing pool" may take place, and the period during which such tests may be carried out. They require the athletes

---

63 *National Federation of Sportspersons* (n 63) para 11
64 Ibid
65 Ibid (n 60) para 12

in question, in view of the demands of efforts to combat doping, to provide accurate and up-to-date information on their whereabouts for the purposes of organising tests, including unannounced tests, with a view to the effective detection of the use of doping substances, which can be detected only for a short time after being taken despite having lasting effects. Hence, Articles 3 and 7 of the impugned order, which do not hamper athletes' freedom of movement, interfere with their right to respect for their private and family life as guaranteed by Article 8, and with individual freedoms, only to the extent that is necessary and proportionate to the general-interest aims pursued by efforts to combat doping, namely to protect athletes' health and to ensure fair and ethical sporting competitions. In any event, the order under challenge also complies with the provisions of the International Convention against Doping in Sport, which do not have direct effect.

Athletes whose names feature on the list of elite sportsmen and women or the list of promising young athletes, which include amateur athletes and licensed professionals who may be required to notify their whereabouts with a view to anti-doping tests, are not in the same situation as other athletes, in view of the level at which they compete and the greater risk of doping such competition may entail. Likewise, athletes who have been the subject of disciplinary sanctions for doping during the past three years are not in the same situation as other athletes. Furthermore, athletes belonging to the "testing pool" are not in the same situation as persons in other professions and may therefore be made subject to special doping control measures without the principle of equality being breached.[66]

Being aggrieved, the applicants made their challenge before the ECHR by taking recourse to Article 34 of the Convention for the Protection of Human Rights and Fundamental Freedoms.[67] The ECHR perused the arguments and held that

the whereabouts requirement constitutes interference with the applicants' exercise of their rights under the first paragraph of Article 8. Such interference will be in breach of Article 8 unless it is "in accordance with the law," pursues one or more of the legitimate aims under the second paragraph of that Article and is "necessary in a democratic society" in order to achieve the aim or aims concerned.[68]

---

66 Ibid
67 Council of Europe, "Convention for the Protection of Human Rights and Fundamental Freedoms as Amended by Protocols No. 11 and No. 14" Article 34 [Article 34 – Individual applications The Court may receive applications from any person, non-governmental organization or group of individuals claiming to be the victim of a violation by one of the High Contracting Parties of the rights set forth in the Convention or the protocols thereto. The High Contracting Parties undertake not to hinder in any way the effective exercise of this right.]
68 *National Federation of Sportspersons* (n 61) para 159

The ECHR then went on to hold that

> In view of the precise and detailed provisions of this instrument, which was adopted by a State authority in accordance with the provisions of the WADC, the Court considers that it allows licensed athletes, with the support of a coach, to regulate their conduct and be afforded sufficient protection against arbitrariness.
>
> In sum, the interference in question was "in accordance with the law" within the meaning of Article 8 § 2 of the Convention.[69]

Importantly, the ECHR upheld that the main aim of the whereabouts requirement is to protect the health of the athletes. ECHR holds that

> As regards the first aim referred to, namely the protection of "health," the Court observes, like the Government, that this aim is enshrined in the relevant international instruments and that all the evidence in the file is consistent with that aim. The Council of Europe Convention (see paragraph 40 above), the WADC (see paragraph 45 above), the UNESCO Convention (see paragraph 53 above) and the Sports Code (see paragraph 57 above) are unanimous in presenting efforts to combat doping as a health concern which the sporting world is seeking to address (see paragraphs 171 to 177 below). Consequently, the Court accepts that the whereabouts requirement is designed to address issues concerning "health," within the meaning of the second paragraph of Article 8, with regard to both professional and amateur athletes and with a particular focus on young people.[70]

Thus, ECHR puts health as the primary aim of all anti-doping measures. Protection of morality and fair play and equal opportunity are treated by the ECHR as the second aim of the WADA Code and other international instruments on anti-doping.[71] Proceeding further with the health argument as the most important goal of the WADA Code and other anti-doping instruments, the ECHR held that

> doping represents a real threat to athletes' physical and mental health. The Court does not rule out the possibility, as asserted by the applicants, that athletes' health may be harmed by factors unconnected to the taking of doping agents, in view of the intensity and high level of competitions. It notes in that connection the constant pressure to which some of them are subjected and observes that the relevant reports advocate regulating the number of competition fixtures (see paragraphs 74 and 88 above). However, the Court

69 Ibid para 162–163
70 Ibid para 165
71 Ibid para 166

regards the demanding nature of top-level sporting competitions as a further reason to protect the health of those taking part against the dangers inherent in doping, rather than as a reason to reduce efforts to combat the practice.

Furthermore, while action to combat doping is a public-health issue in professional sport . . . it concerns all athletes.[72]

Thus the ECHR concluded that

the Court is satisfied that the health and public-health considerations at stake in the present case, and the legitimate ethical concerns in that regard . . . constitute a decisive argument for the necessity of the interference resulting from the impugned whereabouts requirement.[73]

Reiterating the urgency to protect the health of the athlete the ECHR dismissed the challenge posed by the applicants by reiterating that

The Court does not underestimate the impact of the whereabouts requirements on the applicants' private lives. Nevertheless, the general interest considerations that make them necessary are particularly important and, in the Court's view, justify the restrictions on the applicants' rights. . . . Reducing or removing the requirements of which the applicants complain would be liable to increase the dangers of doping to their health and that of the entire sporting community, and would run counter to the European and international consensus on the need for unannounced testing.[74]

WADA was quick to take note of the ECHR emphasis on health as the primary justification for the anti-doping regime. As is evident from the draft of the 2021 WADA Code, WADA has changed the order in which the values of sport are listed. The values, as listed by WADA, encompass what is called the "spirit of sport." Health has been pushed up the order and leads the pack.[75] This change under the pressure of the ECHR judgement is remarkable. Further, the explanation to the "Fundamental rationale for the World Anti-Doping Code" is proposed to be amended in the draft in the following way viz. "Doping is fundamentally contrary to the spirit of sport. And the protection of Athletes' health and right to compete on a doping free level playing field as set forth in the Anti-Doping Charter of Athletes' Rights."[76] The health argument has been given by many who argue for a radical revision of WADA's philosophy. The argument

72 Ibid (n 60) 175
73 Ibid para 177
74 Ibid para 191
75 WADA, "World Anti-Doping Code 2021" *The Draft* www.wada-ama.org/sites/default/files/2018_06_04_code_draft_version_0.1.pdf (accessed 6 December 2018)
76 Ibid

questions the spirit of sport logic and the right to participate on a level playing field. As noted, there is no level play between elite and non-elite developing country athletes. Sports are inherently unequal, with skilled people having a better chance of winning. Developed country athletes always have a comparative advantage against developing country athletes in terms of resources and facilities available. Hence, it's time to discard the argument of a level playing field to justify the current anti-doping system. Given that WADA has conceded to health arguments as the most important aim for the 2021 Code, we might as well proceed further. As the radical libertarians are arguing, all the athletes should be permitted the use of PEDs. The only caveat being that those which are harmful to health should be included in the Prohibited List. The focus therefore shifts from performance enhancement to health protection. This will cut down on the logistical and financial pressure currently weighing upon the anti-doping agencies, including WADA.[77]

The other structural reform that has been suggested by many is that WADA should be completely outside the purview of nations as well as the IOC and its members. Hence, the governing body of WADA should be headed by independent persons having no hidden or other agendas. These independent persons can then implement WADA in an objective and transparent manner. All the stakeholders who are interested in effective doping enforcement are expected to fund WADA. Funding should be done as part of the international commitment to implement the WADA Code. In fact, funding obligations should be part and parcel of WADA compliance. However, funding partners should not be allowed to influence WADA's decision-making power. Having independent persons heading WADA will protect against any exercise of such influence. In addition, decision-making power needs to be shifted from sports federations and governments to a committee of independent persons having expertise in various aspects of sports. These changes are suggested in the composition of two of the most powerful bodies of WADA viz. the WADA's Foundation Board and WADA's Executive Board. A new body termed the WADA Governance and Nominations Committee will be created, composed of independent persons, to oversee the functioning of the WADA Foundation Board and Executive Committee.[78] These reforms pre-suppose that funds will be provided by the international community without seeking a stake in the WADA pie. It pre-supposes that the governments will let go of power and act as benign spectators. In short, these proposals are radical and far-reaching. However, with the post Russian scandal developments one can only hope that WADA does become fit for the purpose.

77 Bengt Kayser, Alexandre Mauron and Andy Miah, "Current Anti-Doping Policy: A Critical Appraisal" BMC Medical Ehtics (2007) https://bmcmedethics.biomedcentral.com/articles/10.1186/1472-6939-8-2#Sec2 (accessed 6 December 2018)
78 Ali Jawad, "The Alternative: Reforming WADA's Governance for a New Anti-Doping Age" (2018) http://athletesforcleansport.com/wp-content/uploads/2018/10/The-Alternative-Reforming-WADAs-Governance-for-a-new-Anti-Doping-Age.pdf (accessed 6 December 2018)

Conclusion

There has been a huge outcry over WADA's decision to reinstate RUSADA, as mentioned earlier. This outcry is justified in view of the blatant infractions of the WADA Code. However, the outcry has also led to a re-assertion of hope.[79] Hope not to let go of WADA, and to continue to believe that WADA is the best bet one has. The non-elite developing country athlete understands that unless resources are provided and technological assistance is given, competing with First World athletes is difficult, if not impossible. The non-elite developing country athlete therefore has no reason to rejoice or feel hopeful for any wide-ranging reforms. The ongoing WADA Code revision 2021 does not create space for any alternative thought process. Barring a cosmetic change being made to the rationale for WADA Code, on paper there is nothing that inspires confidence. As the set of questions framed by WADA indicates, the status quo will be maintained. We will continue to be governed by the rationale of spirit of sport. The applicability of strict liability will continue to be there. The presumption of innocence will not benefit the athletes. The governing bodies are not going to be accountable for shoddy handling of arbitration proceedings and evidence gathering. The non-elite athlete will be vulnerable to the whims and facies of the government and NADA and WADA. In such a scenario, unless there is an assertion of the collective will of all the stakeholders to uphold the essence of anti-doping regime and be empathetic to the cause of the non-elite athlete, the way forward is bleak.[80] For WADA to be fit for the purpose, it has to not only ensure effective enforcement of the anti-doping regime but also has to co-opt the viewpoint of the non-elite developing country athlete and become the document of change.

Bibliography

AFP/Bicycling.com, "Chris Froome Cleared in Doping Probe, Allowed to Race in Tour de France the Uci's Decision Clears Froome to Go for a Historic Fifth Tour Win" *Bicycling* (2018) www.bicycling.com/news/a22019610/chris-froome-cleared-doping/ (accessed 5 December 2018)

Australian Sports Anti-Doping Agency, "Organisational Structure" www.asada.gov.au/sites/default/files/Org%20structure.pdf?v=1466401128 (accessed 5 December 2018)

Chougule, A. L. I. "BCCI Must Go Easy on Muscle-flexing" *The Free Press Journal* (New Delhi, 12 May 2017) www.freepressjournal.in/editorspick/ali-chougule-bcci-must-go-easy-on-muscle-flexing/1066668 (accessed 6 December 2018)

---

79 Institute of National Anti-Doping Organizations, "International Anti-Doping Leaders Stand United with International Athlete Community in Calling for Meaningful Reform of WADA Governance" *Media Release* (2018) www.inado.org/fileadmin/user_upload/_temp_/2018_Oct._NADO_Leaders_Meeting_in_Paris.pdf (accessed 6 December 2018)

80 Owen Gibson, "A Truly Independent Wada Should Have the Power to Sanction Sports and Nations" *The Guardian* (London, 11 November 2015)

Council of Europe, "Convention for the Protection of Human Rights and Fundamental Freedoms as amended by Protocols No. 11 and No. 14" Article 34

Cycling Independent Reform Commission, Report to the President of the Union Cycliste Internationale (2015) *Lausanne* 16 https://s27394.pcdn.co/wp-content/uploads/2015/03/CIRC-Report-2015.pdf (accessed 3 December 2018)

Der Spiegel Staff, "Doping Irregularities Ramos, Ronaldo and the Controllers" *Spiegel Online* (Berlin, 23 November 2018) www.spiegel.de/international/world/football-leaks-doping-tests-and-real-madrid-a-1240035.html (accessed 4 December 2018)

Dyer, Bryce, "The Controversy of Sports Technology: A Systematic Review" (2015) www.ncbi.nlm.nih.gov/pmc/articles/PMC4575312/ (accessed 4 December 2018)

European Convention on Human Rights, Article 8 www.echr.coe.int/Documents/Convention_ENG.pdf (accessed 7 December 2018)

Gibson, Owen, "A Truly Independent Wada Should Have the Power to Sanction Sports and Nations" *The Guardian* (London, 11 November 2015)

Inside UCI, "UCI Statement on Anti-Doping Proceedings Involving Mr Christopher Froome" (2018) www.uci.org/inside-uci/press-releases/uci-statement-on-anti-doping-proceedings-involving-mr-christopher-froome (accessed 5 December 2018)

Institute of National Anti-Doping Organizations, "International Anti-Doping Leaders Stand United with International Athlete Community in Calling for Meaningful Reform of WADA Governance" (2018) www.inado.org/fileadmin/user_upload/_temp_/2018_Oct._NADO_Leaders_Meeting_in_Paris.pdf (accessed 6 December 2018)

Jawad, Ali, "The Alternative: Reforming WADA's Governance for a New Anti-Doping Age" (2018) http://athletesforcleansport.com/wp-content/uploads/2018/10/The-Alternative-Reforming-WADAs-Governance-for-a-new-Anti-Doping-Age.pdf (accessed 6 December 2018)

Kayser, Bengt, Alexandre Mauron and Andy Miah, "Current Anti-Doping Policy: A Critical Appraisal" BMC *Medical Ehtics* (2007) https://bmcmedethics.biomedcentral.com/articles/10.1186/1472-6939-8-2#Sec2 (accessed 6 December 2018)

"Lance Armstrong Stripped of All Seven Tour de France Wins by UCI" BBC (London, 22 October 2012) www.bbc.com/sport/cycling/20008520 (accessed 5 December 2018)

Lindsey, Joe, "The Problem with Clearing Chris Froome the Uci's Decision Shows There Are Two Sets of Rules in Cycling: One for Rich Superstars, and One for Everyone Else" *Bicycling* (2018) www.bicycling.com/racing/a22038157/uci-chris-froome-doping/ (accessed 5 December 2018)

NADA, "WADA Report on Doping Violations: India Improves its Global Anti-Doping Record" (2018) www.nadaindia.org/upload_file/document/1525277616.pdf (accessed 6 December 2018)

Nathanson, Patrick and Jack Skelton, "Chris Froome: UCI President Says Team Sky's Wealth Helped Them Fight Case in Way Other Teams Could Not" BBC *Sport* (London, 6 July 2018) www.bbc.com/sport/cycling/44739022 (accessed 5 December 2018)

National Federation of Sportspersons' Associations and Unions (FNASS) and Others v. France ECHR (Fifth Section) 2018 https://hudoc.echr.coe.int/eng#{%22itemid%22:[%22001-180442%22]} (accessed 6 December 2018)

SI WIRE, "Ex-IAAF President Lamine Diack Confesses to Asking Russia for Money" *Sports Illustrated* (2015) www.si.com/more-sports/2015/12/18/iaaf-corruption-lamine-diack-confession-russian-doping-scandal-bribe (accessed 5 December 2018)

TNN, "BCCI Turns Down Wada's Demand to Test Cricketers" *The Times of India Sports* (New Delhi, 11 November 2017) https://timesofindia.indiatimes.com/sports/cricket/news/bcci-turns-down-wadas-demand-to-test-cricketers/articleshow/61601043.cms (accessed 4 December 2018)

United States Anti-Doping Agency, "United States Anti-Doping Agency, Claimant, v. Lance Armstrong, Respondent-Reasoned Decision of the United States Anti-Doping Agency on Disqualification and Ineligibility" (2012) Report on Proceedings Under the World Anti-Doping Code and the Usada Protocol

WADA, 2009

WADA, 2015 Code

WADA, "2021 World Anti-Doping Code Review: Questions to Discuss and Consider" As Per the Decision Taken by the WADA Foundation Board on 16 November 2017 in Seoul, Korea www.wada-ama.org/sites/default/files/2021codereview_questions.pdf (accessed 5 December 2018)

WADA, "WADA Clarifies Facts Regarding UCI Decision on Christopher Froome" (2018) www.wada-ama.org/en/media/news/2018-07/wada-clarifies-facts-regarding-uci-decision-on-christopher-froome (accessed 5 December 2018)

WADA, "World Anti-Doping Code 2021" *The Draft* www.wada-ama.org/sites/default/files/2018_06_04_code_draft_version_0.1.pdf (accessed 6 December 2018)

World Anti-Doping Code, "International Standard-Prohibited List" 1 January 2018 www.wada-ama.org/sites/default/files/prohibited_list_2018_en.pdf (accessed 6 December 2018)

Xataka, "Everything about technological doping in cycling" *Medium* (2015) https://medium.com/@Xataka/everything-about-technological-doping-in-cycling-78c7fd1fe3f (accessed 5 December 2018)

Chapter 6

Conclusions

Right from the beginning of its journey, WADA and its predecessor, the IOC Medical Commission, authored an anti-doping narrative that ignores the realities of professionalism. That professionals need to earn a livelihood was completely ignored. Sport was elevated to the status of pure and sacred. Mere mortals were not supposed to spoil it. Hence the justification of prohibiting PEDs is more ethical than practical. The current anti-doping narrative ignores the past, imagines the present as ideal and does not acknowledge the challenges of the future. The experiences of the discourse leading to the establishment of WADA reveal a process of self-denial. The spirit-of-sport argument fuels the anti-doping narrative and creates a scenario where there are no alternative discussions. This denial of the realities has resulted in the intervention of the government and public authorities. WADA was created to instill accountability in the system and assure athletes that there would be genuine cases taken up as that of ADRVs. The problem is that the intrusions of governments have not improved the scenario. On the contrary, WADA governance appears more as a saga of power play than a genuine concern for athletes. In this quagmire the worst sufferers, as always, are the athletes. The Russian scandal proves that it's a long way to proper implementation of the WADA Code. The Russian scandal is the biggest challenge that WADA has faced to date and has led to existential questions for WADA. These questions, however, have been made murkier with the ambivalence of the anti-doping agency and other authorities. This ambivalence is evident in the response to the Russian scandal that highlighted the differences amongst the various sports authorities.

What WADA did on 20 September 2018 was an encore of the IOC's performance on 28 February 2018. On that day the IOC lifted the ban on the Russian Olympic Committee. This was in compliance with the decision of the IOC Executive Board taken on 25 February 2018. The IOC's laxity towards Russia is evident from the fact that during the 2018 Olympic Winter Games in Pyeongchang two athletes of the OAR tested positive for doping. Despite such infractions, the IOC lifted the ban on the ROC. The maximum punishment it awarded to the ROC for the latest doping positives was to ban them from the Closing Ceremony. Thus, two of the leading flag-bearers of anti-doping enforcement viz.

WADA and IOC have welcomed back Russia. The other powerful International Sports Federation, the Fédération Internationale de Football Association (FIFA), has been equally lax towards Russia. FIFA ignored the hue and cry over the Russian doping scandal and went along with the 2018 FIFA World Cup in Russia. In this scenario, the power of the Russian State seems to overwhelm any will to deal with the issue of state-sponsored doping. Further as the CAS decisions reveal, the IOC's handling of the Russian doping cases was clumsy to say the least. Given the realities of such blatant favouritism towards a powerful elite sports nation, one really has no hope for the developing country athletes. This also sends a message that the powerful and rich can get away with doping. The series of latest controversies, post the Russian scandal, affirms this concern. It appears that the troika of WADA, IOC and the International Federations are working hard to preserve the hegemony of the star athletes, the powerful nations and corporate commercial interests. On 4 December 2018, the IAAF decided not to reinstate Russian Athletics (RusAF). The IAAF has set two condition precedent for the reinstatement of RusAF which are:

1   The IAAF be given *"all of the data and access to the samples that it needs to determine which of the Russian athletes in the LIMS database have a case to answer for breach of the IAAF anti-doping rules. The IAAF Council was clear that Russian athletes cannot return to international competition unconditionally until that issue is resolved one way or the other."*
2   That RusAF must pay up for all the costs *"incurred in the work of the Taskforce and in bringing or defending Russian cases at CAS. The IAAF Council was clear that this debt must be settled for reinstatement to occur; it is not fair to ask the IAAF and its other members to continue to carry these costs."*

Can the IAAF decision be regarded as a beacon of hope? Or is it a PR gimmick to bolster the IAAF's image? One will await the decision's impact, but there is a sense that such a one-off approach does not augur well for the world of sports. Consequentially, the stringent provision within the WADA Code appears to be meant to promote the interests of the elite sportspersons and their nations. Stringency has increased at the cost of the non-elite athletes. On the contrary, the elite get to hire the best scientists and lawyers and win their way through CAS arbitration. A review of the various aspects of the current anti-doping regime under the WADA Code reveals a lot. To be precise, the incorporation of the strict liability principle in the Code strengthens the cause of the elites more than the non-elite/developing country athletes. The doctrine imposes unrealistic expectations on them in view of the circumstances of a non-elite/developing country athlete. The Code has incorporated provisions to soften the rigour of the doctrine and develop a modified form of strict liability. However, it has softened the rigour to the extent of giving the athlete a chance to rebut the presumption of an anti-doping rule violation. On the failure of the athlete to rebut the presumption of an ADRV, the result of the event is automatically disqualified. And the rebuttal is excessively tough since one has to challenge the entire system and result management process. Alternatively, one has to show TUE, which is equally tough to obtain. Thus, the amount of resources needed to challenge ADRV is likely to dissuade non-elite/developing country athletes from pursuing the matter. These inbuilt constraints thus tend to make the WADA Code an elitist doctrine. The advantage of the elite gets highlighted day in day out.

Such a thing happened on 27 February 2018 when the UK Parliament published a report on doping in sport. Apart from everything else, what the report revealed was the abuse of TUEs for performance enhancement. The sport in respect of which this finding was published was British Cycling. The star performer whose TUE was under scrutiny was Sir Bradley Wiggins. The Committee concluded that TUEs were being abused for gaining performance enhancement. These findings exemplify the advantages that the elite take or are in a position to take under the current anti-doping regime. However, as one saw in the case of developing countries like Kenya and India, the non-elite athletes are nowhere near abusing the system. They don't even have the means to abuse, and that is precisely the reason why they get caught so easily. The divide between the elite and the non-elite cannot be abridged with system changes. On the contrary, every new stringency in the WADA Code affects the rights of the non-elite to be treated fairly. And this affects their ability to use the existing processes to prove their innocence. The scrutiny of CAS decisions reveals how poorly the arguments are made. There is no support system to help athletes once they are caught. And there is no system to instill accountability amongst anti-doping agencies. In view of these realities, WADA has not yet done anything to help assuage feelings as to the future of the anti-doping system.

There has been a huge outcry over WADA's decision to reinstate RUSADA, as mentioned earlier. This outcry is justified in view of the blatant infractions of the WADA Code. However, the outcry has also led to a re-assertion of hope. Hope not to let go of WADA, and to continue to believe that WADA is the best bet one has. The non-elite developing country athlete understands that unless resources are provided and technological assistance is given, competing with First World athletes is difficult, if not impossible. Therefore, the non-elite developing country athlete has no reason to either rejoice or feel hopeful for any wide-ranging reforms. The ongoing 2021 ADA Code revision does not create space for any alternative thought process. Barring a cosmetic change being made to the rationale for WADA Code, there is nothing on paper that inspires confidence. As the set of questions framed by WADA indicates, the status quo will be maintained. We will continue to be governed by the rationale of spirit of sport. The applicability of strict liability will continue to be there. The presumption of innocence will not benefit the athletes. The governing bodies will not be accountable for shoddy handling of arbitration proceedings and evidence gathering. The non-elite athlete will be vulnerable to the whims and facies of the government and NADA and WADA. In such a scenario unless there is an assertion of the collective will of all the stakeholders to uphold the essence of the anti-doping regime and to be empathetic to the cause of the non-elite athlete, the way forward is bleak. For WADA to be fit for the purpose it must not only ensure effective enforcement of the anti-doping regime but also co-opt the viewpoint of the non-elite developing country athlete and become the document of change.

Index